HIV Infection and AIDS

Siobhan M. Murphy FRCPI
Consultant Physician
Department of Genitourinary Medicine
The Patrick Clements Clinic
Central Middlesex Hospital NHS Trust
London

Gary Brook MD FRCP
Consultant Physician
Department of Genitourinary Medicine
The Patrick Clements Clinic
Central Middlesex Hospital NHS Trust
London

Martin A. Birchall MD (Cantab)
Reader in Head and Neck Surgery
Honorary Consultant in Otolaryngology
University of Bristol and Southmead Hospital
Bristol

D0967890

SECOND EDITION

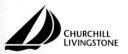

CHURCHILL
LIVINGSTONE

EDINBURGH LONDON NEW YORK PHILADELPHIA ST LOUIS SYDNEY
TORONTO 2000

CHURCHILL LIVINGSTONE
An imprint of Harcourt Publishers Limited

© Harcourt Publishers Limited 2000
© Illustrations
M. I. G. Chelsea and Westminster Hospital:
Figures 4, 8, 11, 28, 29, 36, 40, 41, 42, 43, 44, 45,
46, 51, 52, 53, 55, 56, 57, 58, 60, 62, 63, 66, 67, 68,
69, 70, 72, 73, 75, 80, 83, 85, 95, 100, 106, 110
Western Ophthalmic Hospital: Figures 111, 112,
113, 114

First published as Colour Guide: HIV Infection and
AIDS 1992
Second Colour Guide edition 2000

ISBN 0443 06168 8

British Library Cataloguing in Publication Data
A catalogue record for this book is available from
the British Library

Library of Congress Cataloging in Publication Data
A catalog record for this book is available from
the Library of Congress

Note
Medical knowledge is constantly
changing. As new information
becomes available, changes in
treatment, procedures, equipment
and the use of drugs become
necessary. The authors and the
publishers have, as far as it is
possible, taken care to ensure
that the information given in this
text is accurate and up-to-date.
However, readers are strongly
advised to confirm that the
information, especially with
regard to drug usage, complies
with the latest legislation and
standards of practice.

The
publisher's
policy is to use
**paper manufactured
from sustainable forests**

Printed in China
SWTC/01

Commissioning Editor:
Michael Parkinson
Project Development Manager:
Siân Jarman
Project Manager: Nancy Arnott
Design Direction: Erik Bigland

Preface

It is now almost a decade since the first edition of *HIV Infection and AIDS* was written. The clinical problem of HIV infection continues to represent one of the biggest challenges facing health service workers. However, major advances in the diagnosis and treatment of HIV infection with highly active antiretroviral therapy (HAART) have been made. The impact on the developed world of these developments are reflected by a marked drop in both the number of patients dying from AIDS and the number of HIV-infected patients requiring treatment in hospital. Sadly, at the current time, because HAART is very expensive, these medications are not available generally in those parts of the world where the prevalence of HIV is highest.

This edition has been re-organized by adding some completely new chapters and rewriting and updating many of the previous chapters. There are new symptom-based chapters on fever and constitutional symptoms and this edition also includes some system-based topics, for example, musculoskeletal problems and the urogenital system. The final chapter, entitled 'Approaches to Therapy', has been completely rewritten to reflect the introduction of HAART and how it has changed the course of HIV disease. A new chapter on pregnancy has been included, to reflect the huge advances in the care of the pregnant mother in reducing mother-to-child transmission of HIV. Other chapters which have been substantially changed include those on epidemiology, the diagnosis of HIV infection and the classification of HIV-related disease.

This book, as before, is not intended to be a comprehensive text book on HIV or AIDS medicine, but rather to give an insight into some of the more common clinical features of HIV infection and AIDS and of the recent changes and advances in treatment. The area of HIV medicine is continuously being researched and under review and hence many of the statements in this edition are likely to change over time.

London   S. M. M.
2000   G. B.
                                                           M. A. B.

Acknowledgements

We are indebted to all the individuals who provided slides from their personal collections in preparing the second edition. Many of the illustrations from the first edition are re-used here. These were contributed generously by Dr C. Amerasinghe, Abbott Diagnostics Ltd, Dr G. Bellingham, Blackwell Scientific Publications, Dr C. Conlon, Dr P. Dickman, Miss C. Donegan, Dr A. Hines, Dr J. M. Jacobs, Dr O. Lau, Dr R. Logan, Dr J. Leonard, Dr G. Mason, Mr C. Migdal, Dr F. Moss, Dr M. McCarthy, Dr B. Peters, Mr N. Stafford, Dr F. Scaravelli, Dr K. Suvarna, Mr M. Savage, Dr J. Selles, Mr D. Simmons, Dr S. Soucek, Dr S. Stewart, Mr A. Tanner, Dr D. Tomlinson, Dr J. Wyner, Dr S. Walters, Westway Graphics and Wolfe Publishing Ltd. We are indebted to The Medical Illustration Department, at Chelsea and Westminster Hospital, for permission to use slides from their collections.

For this second edition, additional pictures and advice have generously been contributed by Dr C. Amerasinghe, Dr A. Hines, Dr I. Knockler, Dr F. Chen and Dr T. Chowdhury and the right to reproduce Figure 1 is gratefully acknowledged to UNAIDS publications on www.unaids.org

Contents

1 / History and epidemiology of HIV and AIDS

History of AIDS

The first cases of the acquired immune deficiency syndrome (AIDS) were reported in June 1981, when five cases of *Pneumocystis carinii* pneumonia (PCP) in homosexual men in California, USA were described. One month later, 26 cases of unusually aggressive Kaposi's sarcoma (KS) in homosexual men, some of whom also had PCP, were reported in New York, USA. By the end of 1982, it was clear that an outbreak of a new acquired immune deficiency syndrome had occurred. In 1984, the transmissible agent was identified and finally named as human immunodeficiency virus type 1 (HIV-1). In 1985, a second human immunodeficiency virus (HIV-2) was identified in western Africa, which gave rise to a clinically similar disease.

There are different strains of HIV-1 known as 'subtypes' or 'clades' and designated A to H. Subtype B is the most common strain in the UK and USA, subtype A in Africa and subtype E in Thailand.

Epidemiology of HIV

By the end of 1997, the World Health Organisation (WHO) estimated that over 30 million people were infected with HIV worldwide. Of these over 1 million were children. If current trends continue, in the year 2000, more than 40 million people may be living with HIV.

The epidemiological pattern has changed. In the west in the early years, the disease was mainly confined to homosexual men, i.v. drug users and recipients of blood products. By the late 1980s, it was clear that there was a high prevalence of AIDS in sub-Saharan Africa, where it was predominantly heterosexually spread. In the developed world, homosexual men still comprise the largest infected group.

The worldwide epidemic of HIV infection is evolving into a mainly heterosexually transmitted disease of the developing world and of poor and marginalized populations in the industrialized world (Fig. 1).

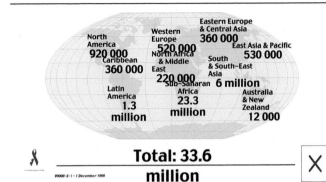

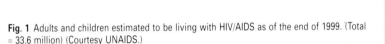

Fig. 1 Adults and children estimated to be living with HIV/AIDS as of the end of 1999. (Total = 33.6 million) (Courtesy UNAIDS.)

Sub-Saharan Africa is still the area worst affected by HIV-1. It is almost exclusively a heterosexually spread disease with almost equal incidence in men and women; children often acquire their infection from their mothers. The reasons for the rapid spread on the African continent are multiple, including:

1. Migration of workers from rural to urban areas where HIV prevalence is high, and their subsequent return to the rural areas
2. Population shifts because of war
3. Poor availability of primary care for the treatment of sexually transmitted infections, in particular ulcerative disease, which predispose to HIV transmission
4. Prostitution, particularly along major highways
5. Unavailability of barrier method of contraception
6. Mother-to-child transmission rates are high (see Ch. 19)
7. More frequent use of blood transfusions without prior HIV screening.

In Africa the epidemic has also been changing over time. Central and eastern Africa were affected in the late 1970s and current estimates are that up to 36% of the total population in eastern Africa is now infected. However, massive health education and HIV-prevention programmes appear to be having positive effects as the epidemic is plateauing in some countries, e.g. Uganda. South Africa has seen a recent explosive epidemic of the infection. In western Africa, the area most densely affected is the Ivory Coast and surrounding countries with the huge migrations for work. HIV-2 is also found in most western African countries, but the rate of spread is not as fast as that of HIV-1.

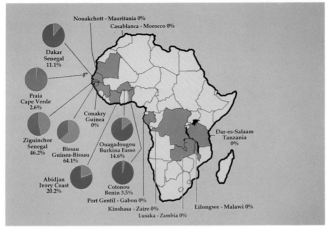

Fig. 2 Distribution of HIV-2 in Africa. The pie charts show the proportions of population infected in specific areas.

2 / Classification of HIV-related disease

Early classification

In 1982 and subsequently in 1985 and 1987, the American Centers for Disease Control (CDC) introduced a case definition for AIDS, as a cluster of conditions seen in the early part of the HIV outbreak. This definition consisted of a list of infections, malignancies and constitutional illness that signified immunodeficiency in these previously healthy people. The American definition subsequently included a low CD4+ lymphocyte count as an AIDS-defining event, although this was not uniformly accepted elsewhere, including the UK. In 1984, other terms used to describe HIV-related illness (not amounting to full-blown AIDS) came into use, including the AIDS-related complex (ARC), seroconversion illness and persistent generalised lymphadenopathy. This classification has been superseded by other more clinically relevant schemes but the AIDS definition has been retained as an epidemiological tool to describe the HIV epidemic. All patients meeting the AIDS case definition are still reported to the national epidemiological bodies such as the Communicable Disease Surveillance Centre for England and Wales or the Communicable Disease Unit, Ruchill, Glasgow (Scotland).

Current classification

Given the importance of plasma viral load and blood CD4+ lymphocyte measurements as prognostic tools (see Ch. 5), it is more usual to refer to the illness simply in terms of symptomatic or asymptomatic disease. The CDC classification of HIV-related conditions still has some relevance as it broadly describes symptomatic disease as it relates to declining immune competence (Table 1). ➡

Table 1 Centers for Disease Control (CDC) classification of HIV-related disease (1986)

Stage	Description
I	Acute infection (seroconversion illness)
II	Asymptomatic infection
III	Persistent generalized lymphadenopathy
IV	Symptomatic disease:

A. Constitutional disease (e.g. HIV Wasting syndrome)

B. Neurological disease (e.g. mononeuritis, myelopathy)

C. Infections indicative of a defect in cell-mediated immunity
   1. AIDS-defining infections (e.g. *Pneumocystis carinii* pneumonitis, CMV retinitis, cryptococcal meningitis etc.)
   2. Non-AIDS defining infections (e.g. oral candidiasis, single episode of bacterial pneumonia, shingles)

D. Malignant disease (e.g. Kaposi's sarcoma, non-Hodgkin's lymphoma)

E. Other conditions (e.g. lymphoid interstitial pneumonitis)

HIV is an RNA virus that uses the enzyme reverse transcriptase to produce DNA from the RNA template, classifying it as a retrovirus. The viral DNA intermediate can become incorporated into the host cell DNA structure, leading to chronic infection of the cell in a form that is undetectable to the immune system. The virus has receptors that attach to the CD4+ protein, allowing the virus to infect all cells with this marker such as T-helper lymphocytes, macrophages, glial cells and dendritic cells. These cells are important components of the human immune system and infection leads to their eventual destruction and therefore loss of ability to fight certain infections and malignancies. The virus reproduces at a very high rate, producing billions of new viruses each day in each infected person and leading to a steady loss of immunity over the years. This progression can be followed by measuring the gradual loss of CD4+ lymphocytes in the blood and the steady rise of plasma HIV–RNA viral load (see Ch. 5). Without treatment, an infected person will progress to severe symptomatic disease and AIDS in an average of 8–10 years, although there is a great deal of variability between people. There is a relationship between the CD4+ lymphocyte ('T-cell') count and the type of problems expected (Table 2).

Table 2. Progress of immunodeficiency: fall in T-cell count and clinical correlates

CD4+ lymphocyte (T-cell) count ($\times 10^6$/L)	Status/complications
>500	Asymptomatic
250–500	Early symptomatic e.g. oral candidiasis, bacterial pneumonia, tuberculosis, seborrhoeic dermatitis
150–250	Moderately immunocompromised/symptomatic e.g. Kaposi's sarcoma, non-Hodgkin's lymphoma
75–150	Severely immuncompromised e.g. *Pneumocystis carinii* pneumonitis, cerebral toxoplasmosis, cryptococcal meningitis, *Mycobacterium avium-intracellulare*
<75	Very severely immunocompromised e.g. cytomegalovirus (retinitis, encephalitis, radiculitis/myelopathy), progressive multifocal leucoencephalopathy (PML)

3 / Transmission of HIV

Distribution

HIV is spread by direct contact with infected blood or bodily fluids with mucous membranes or non-intact skin. HIV has been isolated from most bodily fluids including blood, semen, cervical secretions, breast milk, cerebrospinal fluid, saliva and tears. Of these, blood, semen and cervical secretions are particularly infectious. Saliva, in fact, contains substances inhibitory to HIV replication, and so transmission by this bodily fluid seems less likely. The importance of transmission via heterosexual contact is increasingly emphasized.

Risk factors/ behaviours for HIV acquisition

HIV is spread by:
- Anal or vaginal sexual intercourse
- Transfusion of blood or blood products (this mode of spread is now rare in the developed world as all blood donations are screened for HIV but remains a problem in the developing world (Ch. 1)
- Sharing drug-using equipment, e.g. needles (Fig. 3)
- Inoculation or needlestick injury, usually in the healthcare workplace
- Transmission from mother to child during pregnancy, delivery and breastfeeding. Individuals at highest risk for the acquisition of HIV are listed in Box 1.

Factors affecting transmission rates

Unprotected receptive anal intercourse is the highest-risk sexual behaviour for the acquisition of HIV. In penile–vaginal heterosexual transmission, HIV spreads more easily from man to woman than from woman to man. Sexual transmission is enhanced by the presence of ulcerative and non-ulcerative sexually transmitted infections (STIs) in either partner. Transmission is also enhanced if the infected source has advanced immunodeficiency (characterized by low CD4 T-lymphocyte counts, see Ch. 5) and/or high HIV viral load (see Ch. 19). Triple antiviral therapy reduces HIV viral load and hence patients with non-detectable viral loads will be less infectious.

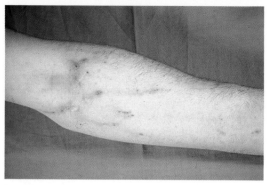

Fig. 3 Puncture marks in young i.v. drug user.

Box 1 Individuals at highest risk of HIV infection

Men who have sex with men
Recipients of infected blood or blood products
I.v. drug users who share needles
Individuals who have sexual intercourse with anyone in the above categories or in
    geographic areas with a high prevalence of HIV
Individuals exposed to the bodily fluids of the above
Children born to mothers in the above groups

4 / Prevention strategies

Safer sex campaigns

The main message is: 'Reduce your number of sexual partners, know your partner's sexual and drug history, and use a condom'. In underdeveloped countries, however, there are major practical and cultural barriers to this approach.

Needle-exchange units

Needle-exchange units provide sterile needles for i.v. drug users, and use the opportunity to educate. Where resources are limited or legislation limits needle exchange, household bleach has been distributed for needle cleaning.

Screening

Screening of donor blood, semen and organs has been employed in wealthier countries since 1985. These remain possible sources of HIV elsewhere.

Strategies to prevent vertical transmission

Vertical transmission from HIV-positive women can be almost eliminated by the use of anti-retroviral agents in pregnancy, usually linked to delivery by Caesarean section and the avoidance of breastfeeding. There is now a very strong argument for 'opt-out' antenatal HIV testing of all pregnant women, especially in areas of high HIV prevalence.

In resource-poor countries, relatively cheap interventions using short-course anti-retrovirals can be effective (an approximate 50% reduction) in preventing vertical transmission, especially if breastfeeding can be safely avoided.

Protection of health care workers

Education around HIV and routes of transmission is vital. This includes safe phlebotomy (Fig. 4), wearing gloves and safe disposal of needles/sharps. Any bodily fluids spilt should be immediately cleaned up with hypochlorite solution. A meticulous operating theatre protocol is essential when dealing with HIV-positive patients (Fig. 5) but many unidentified HIV-positive patients will pass through the theatres. If anti-retrovirals are given soon (ideally <1 h) after the exposure of a health care worker to HIV-containing bodily fluids, it will reduce the risk of infection by 50% or more (post-exposure prophylaxis). Anti-retroviral 'starter packs' should be widely available in most health care settings where sharps injuries are possible.

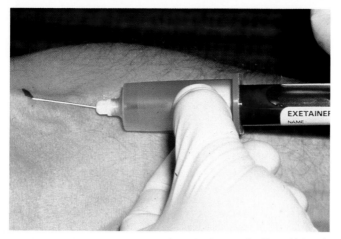

Fig. 4 The use of vacuum-phlebotomy reduces the chances of spillage of infected blood.

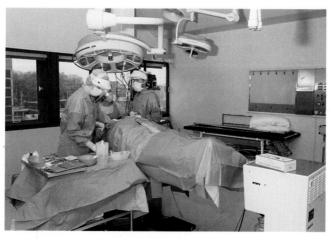

Fig. 5 Operating on a HIV-positive patient: double gloves, disposable gowns, drapes and masks.

5 / Diagnosis of HIV infection

Patients may be diagnosed with HIV infection when they are well or asymptomatic, or when they have clinical signs and symptoms suggestive of HIV infection. Where there is clinical suspicion of HIV infection, confirmatory testing is required. The most commonly used test to diagnose or confirm HIV infection is the HIV antibody test. The seroconversion window period, i.e. the length of time it takes for the HIV antibody (HIV Ab) to develop following infection with the virus is generally taken to be 3 months, although the majority of patients will have developed antibody by 6 weeks. Other tests are utilized in specific circumstances. These other tests include detection of the viral RNA or DNA by polymerase chain reaction (PCR) or culture of virus from peripheral blood mononuclear cells. These latter tests are preferred in situations where the HIV antibody may not yet have developed, e.g. in acute seroconversion illness and in diagnosis of the newborn. Since an infant can carry maternal HIV Ab for up to 18 months, alternative tests are needed for an early diagnosis.

HIV antibody testing

It is standard practise in much of the developed world to undertake HIV pre-test counselling whereby the medical, social, employment and insurance implications of a positive HIV diagnostic test are explained. This is performed by trained health care workers, who also provide psychological support if required after a positive diagnosis. The test is usually performed on a blood sample, however tests for use on urine and saliva have also been developed. ➡

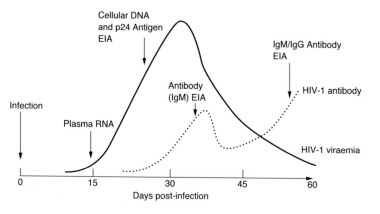

Fig. 6 Graph showing the time when different diagnostic markers can be detected following acute infection. Most modern EIA testing kits for HIV antibody can detect both IgM and IgG.

Tests for HIV antigen and HIV RNA. Antibody appears 3 weeks to 3 months after exposure and may be reliably detected by a variety of commercial kits. Testing for the p24 core antigen is now used less frequently since the development of the molecular biological technique for measuring HIV RNA. Two types of test are currently in general use:

1. reverse transcription (RT) PCR produced by Roche
2. branched DNA (bDNA) produced by Chiron.

These tests amplify genetic particles of the virus and are expressed as RNA copies per ml.

HIV RNA is detectable in the blood around the same time as the HIV p24 core antigen (Figs 6 & 7).

Viral culture and HIV DNA testing. The virus can be cultured from peripheral blood lymphocytes. This test is highly sensitive and specific. Qualitative HIV DNA PCR detects the viral DNA intermediate (see Ch. 2) and is the most commonly used test for diagnosing HIV in infants.

Viral load. The measurement of HIV RNA can be used as a diagnostic test (see above) but its main uses in clinical practice are as follows:

1. As a prognostic indicator, i.e. to assess the rate of progression of the disease to AIDS or death
2. To decide when to start anti-retroviral treatment
3. To monitor the course of the disease
4. To monitor the response to therapy.

In the absence of anti-retroviral treatment, the higher the viral load, the shorter the survival.

T-lymphocytes. The CD4 T-lymphocyte (T-cell) carries the CD4 antigen on its surface. These constitute a subset of the total T (or CD3+) lymphocytes (Box 2). HIV binds itself to the CD4 antigen when entering the lymphocyte (see Fig. 144). The normal CD4 count is between 800 and 1200/cmm. As the patient becomes more immunocompromised the total number of circulating T-cells decreases. The T-cell count is the best available measurement of the patient's immune function. It is measured regularly and used as an indicator as to when to start highly active anti-retroviral therapy (HAART), when to start and/or stop prophylactic medication against opportunistic infections and to monitor the patients immune response to HAART.

ANTIBODY ELISA ASSAY

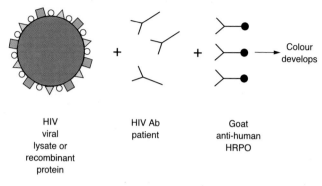

Fig. 7 Mechanism of action of one of the commonly used indirect ELISA tests for HIV antibody.

Box 2 A typical T-lymphocyte (CD3+) subset result. In this patient the CD4+ cells constitute only 14% with an absolute T-cell count of 240/cmm

CD3+ lymphocytes	86%
CD3+ lymphocytes	1.44×10^9
CD4+ lymphocytes	14%
CD4+ lymphocytes	0.24×10^9
CD8+ lymphocytes	68%
CD8+ lymphocytes	1.14×10^9

Clinical features

Acute infection (CDC stage I)

- In about 90% of cases, seroconversion occurs without symptoms.
- The most typical seroconversion illness consists of an acute feverish episode with generalized macular or papular rash, lymphadenopathy, oral and/or genital ulceration and sometimes also tonsillitis – 'glandular-fever-like illness' (Figs 8 & 9).

Other seroconversion syndromes include:

- *Acute, reversible encephalopathy*. This comprises disorientation, loss of memory and altered personality and conscious level.
- *Acute meningoencephalitis* may occur with features of meningeal irritation and drowsiness.
- *Acute myelopathy and neuropathy* has also been reported.

Asymptomatic infection (CDC stage II)

Clinical features

Following the resolution of any seroconversion illness, the great majority of patients enter a phase of asymptomatic infection that can last from 6 months to 20 years or more with a median of about 6 years. This phase can be extended greatly if anti-retroviral therapy is instituted before the onset of symptoms. Patients remain infectious during this period.

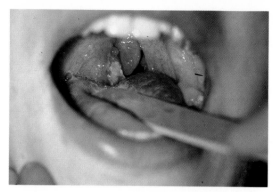

Fig. 8 Acute seroconversion presenting as a glandular-fever-like tonsillitis.

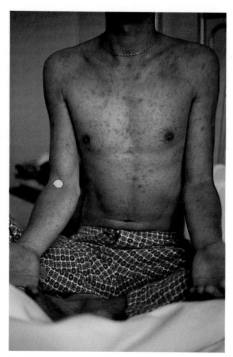

Fig. 9 Papular truncal rash of acute seroconversion illness.

Persistent generalized lymphadenopathy (PGL, CDC stage III)

Definition

A patient having unexplained lymphadenopathy of 3 or more months duration, involving two or more extra-inguinal sites is said to have PGL.

Pathology

Histologically, there is mixed follicular hyperplasia and involution, followed by lymphocyte depletion as disease progresses (Fig. 10).

Clinical features

There is axillary involvement in 98% of cases, and 86% of these involve cervical chains where enlargement is frequently symmetrical (Fig. 11). Splenic and adenoidal enlargement are variably associated. The nodes are usually greater than 1 cm in diameter and may fluctuate in size. PGL is often present for 6 months or more before medical help is sought. There may be constitutional disturbance as above, and occasionally, PGL is associated with a Sjögren-like xerostomia and xerophthalmia.

Differential diagnosis

This includes lymphoma, Kaposi's sarcoma and mycobacteriosis.

Management

In most cases, PGL is asymptomatic and requires no treatment. However, where there is any doubt about the diagnosis, especially markedly asymmetrical lymphadenopathy or constitutional disturbance, further investigation is warranted, including fine-needle aspiration and biopsy.

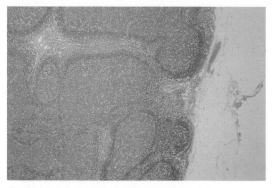

Fig. 10 Lymph node biopsy in PGL: 'geographic' follicular hyperplasia.

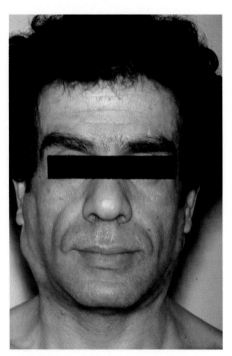

Fig. 11 Bilateral, symmetrical and massive cervical lymphadenopathy in a man with PGL.

Fever is a common presenting symptom in patients with HIV infection. Patients with HIV are prone to all of the usual bacterial and viral infections that may affect a non-HIV-infected patient. A systematic approach is required and must be based on a careful history and clinical examination, looking in particular for clinical evidence of any of the opportunistic infections described elsewhere, and appropriate investigations. These are then interpreted specifically in the light of the patients CD4 T-lymphocyte count and viral load. It is important to remember that constitutional symptoms may arise directly as a result of HIV infection (see Ch. 11).

History

When a patient with HIV presents with a fever, they should be asked how long it has lasted, i.e. days, weeks or months and whether there are associated night sweats and/or weight loss. A systems review may point to a specific problem. Respiratory symptoms, e.g. cough, shortness of breath or sputum production may indicate a respiratory cause of the fever, which can be confirmed by chest X-ray, sputum examination, examination of bronchoalveolar lavage and blood gases (see Ch. 15). Equally the history of gastrointestinal symptoms such as diarrhoea or abdominal pain will lead to investigations of the gastrointestinal tract with stool cultures +/– relevant endoscopic biopsies and perhaps to a diagnosis of an opportunistic infection, e.g. cytomegalovirus (CMV) colitis, salmonella, HIV cholangitis or others as described in Chapter 8. Specific questions with reference to the neurological system may indicate associated headache and/or focal neurological signs, or confusion suggestive of a space-occupying lesion or opportunistic infection such as cryptococcal meningitis as described in Chapter 13. Genitourinary symptoms may lead the investigations to diagnose a urinary tract infection. Remember also that drug fevers can occur.

Box 3 Routine investigations in an HIV-infected patient with fever

Full blood count
Urea electrolytes
Liver function tests
Mid-stream sample of urine
Bacterial and fungal blood culture
Bacterial cultures from any potentially infected site
Chest X-ray
Mycobacterial cultures of blood +/– sputum +/– urine

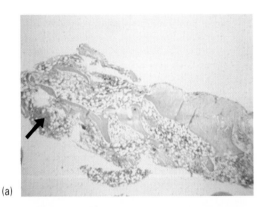

(a)

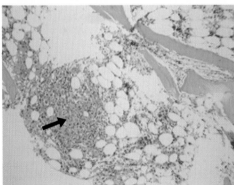

(b)

Fig. 12 (a) Low power magnification. Bone marrow biopsy showing a granuloma. (b) High power magnification. Bone marrow biopsy showing epitheleoid granuloma in keeping with mycobacterium tuberculosis infection.

Routine investigations done in all cases are listed in Box 3. Full blood count may show neutropenia, indicating a secondary bacterial or other infection. If the patient is immunocompromized he/she may not mount a neutrophil response. Liver function tests may show an obstructive pattern indicating an HIV cholangitis and a chest X-ray may indicate a bacterial or opportunistic infection. Bacterial swabs from any potentially infected site, but in particular for urine and blood should be cultured. Blood and sputum cultures should also be taken for mycobacteria, and blood, saliva and urine should be checked for CMV antigen/PCR.

If there are no focal signs diagnoses to be considered include: mycobacterial infection (TB or atypical), lymphoma or cryptococcal infection. It is rare that CMV and disseminated fungal infection other than cryptococcosis are the cause (Box 4).

A bone marrow biopsy and aspirate may be the only test to yield a histological (or culture-proven) diagnosis of mycobacterial disease or other more unusual infections (e.g. histoplasmosis or leishmaniasis), or lymphoma (Figs 12 & 13).

Consider an active search for an occult malignancy, specifically lymphoma, and consider proceeding to abdominal CT or ultrasound scan to look for enlarged lymph nodes that may be biopsied for histology and culture. A CT brain scan and examination of the CSF should be considered in any case of persisting fever. As mentioned above, clinical suspicions and investigation results must be interpreted in the light of the patient's T-cell count, knowing that cryptococcosis, atypical mycobacterial disease and CMV disease occur most commonly when the CD4 T-lymphocyte count is less than 50/ccm (Ch. 2). Lymphoma, although an AIDS-defining illness can occur at any T-cell count.

The treatment of fever is based on the identified cause. Any drug the patient is taking which may be a source of the fever should be stopped. In the absence of an identified cause, a trial of anti-mycobacterial therapy effective against both TB and atypical mycobacterial infection should be considered pending culture results. In addition, anti-retroviral therapy should be commenced or reviewed in the light of the T-cell count and viral load (Ch. 20).

Box 4 Further investigations in an HIV-infected patient with fever

Bone marrow biopsy and aspirate
CMV early antigen testing on blood urine and saliva
Serum cryptococcal antigen
Specific serological tests, e.g. histoplasma complement fixation text
Abdominal ultrasound or computerized tomography (CT) scan
CT brain scan with examination of cerebrospinal fluid (CSF)

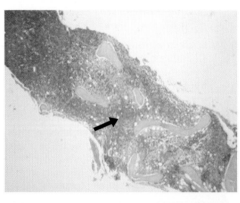

(a)

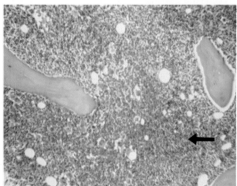

(b)

Fig. 13 (a) Low power magnification. Bone marrow showing infiltration by lymphoma. (b) High power magnification. Lymphoma cells diffusely infiltrating the bone marrow.

Problems of the upper gastrointestinal tract

Oesophageal candidiasis

This is the commonest opportunistic infection of the gastrointestinal tract (GIT) and is an indicator disease for AIDS. The distal oesophagus is the most frequent site.

Pathology

Most infections are by *Candida albicans*, although *C. glabrata* may also occur. The pseudomembranous form, consisting of invasive hyphae with surrounding necrosis, is commoner than the exophytic form. Pseudohyphae do not extend beyond the serosa.

Clinical features

Patients present with retrosternal chest pain and painful dysphagia, or may be asymptomatic. Associated oral candidiasis is common. Like other causes of longstanding chronic inflammation, candidiasis can cause strictures.

Diagnosis

This can be established by barium swallow (Fig. 14) or on endoscopy (Fig. 15). Biopsy or brushings for cytology should be taken to look for invasive pseudohyphae. Culture is not very useful because of the ubiquity of *Candida*.

Differential diagnosis

Similar symptoms can result from other opportunistic infections, e.g. herpes, *Mycobacterium avium-intracellulare* complex (MAC), ulcerating hairy leukoplakia or neoplasia, any of which may coexist.

Management

Oral imidazole antifungal agents such as fluconazole, ketoconazole or itraconazole are usually effective. In very severe cases i.v. amphotericin B may be required. Long-term prophylaxis is not usually required once patients are established on an effective anti-retroviral regimen.

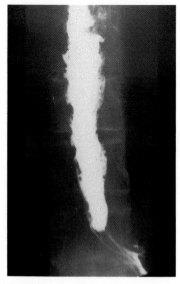

Fig. 14 Barium swallow in oesophageal candidiasis: irregular outline due to swelling and oedema.

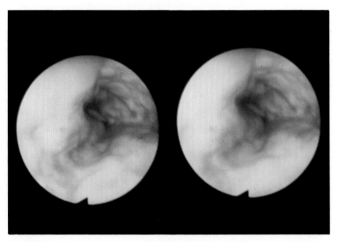

Fig. 15 Severe confluent oesophagitis visible at 23 cm proved to be candidiasis.

CMV oesophagitis

Primary infection with this herpes virus is common in homosexuals and intravenous drug users. Repeated reactivation, shown by reappearance of anti-CMV-IgM and CMV viraemia occurs during HIV infection and may cause disease at any point along the GIT. CMV disease normally only occurs when the CD4 count is less than 100×10^6/l.

Pathology

Infection commences in submucosal cells, where inclusion bodies may be seen. Serpiginous ulcers are characteristic (Figs 16 & 17).

Clinical features

Antifungal-resistant, severe odynophagia is typical. Other evidence of CMV disease, e.g. colitis, may be present.

Diagnosis

The non-specific nature of barium swallow renders endoscopy and biopsy with viral cultures essential.

Management

Virostatic agents (ganciclovir, foscarnet, cidofovir) may lead to long-term remission. Maintenance therapy is not always necessary, especially when a response to anti-retroviral therapy has been seen.

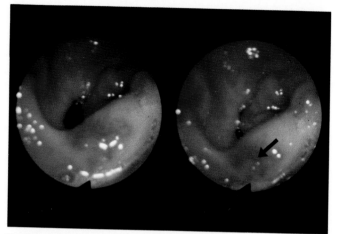

Fig. 16 Endoscopic appearances of CMV oesophagitis.

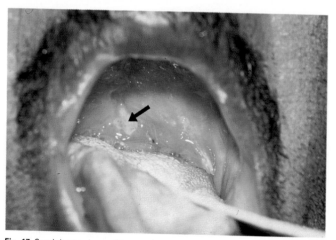

Fig. 17 Serpiginous ulcers of the oropharynx in a patient with CMV oesophagitis.

Herpes simplex oesophagitis

Pathology

Since most adults with AIDS have been infected with HSV types I and/or II, reactivation is common and may affect various parts of the GIT. HSV causes epithelial necrosis. The early vesicles slough, causing circumscribed ulcers (Fig. 18).

Clinical features

Characteristically, there is painful dysphagia. There may be associated pharyngeal ulceration.

Diagnosis

Endoscopic biopsy for histological demonstration of invasive viral infection and viral culture is necessary.

Management

High-dose i.v. acyclovir is required, followed by maintenance oral therapy until there is a response to anti-retroviral treatment. Famciclovir and Penciclovir are also effective.

Problems of the lower gastrointestinal tract

CMV colitis

Clinical features

Up to 10% of AIDS cases are complicated by this. Profuse, liquid diarrhoea, up to 20 stools per day, is characteristic and abdominal pain and weight loss are usual. Rectal bleeding, perforation and toxic dilatation all occur and may be fatal. Untreated, chronic symptoms occur unless punctuated by abdominal catastrophe.

Differential diagnosis

Other infecting organisms, e.g. *Shigella, Clostridium difficile* or MAI, and inflammatory bowel disease may all present in similar fashion to CMV colitis.

Diagnosis

Test for other infectious causes by multiple stool cultures. Sigmoidoscopy with rectal biopsy should be performed. Colonoscopy or flexible sigmoidoscopy is rarely required as involvement of the rectum is almost invariable (Fig. 19).

Management

Acutely, parenteral fluids and nutrition are required. Treatment is with ganciclovir/foscarnet and, subsequently, anti-retrovirals.

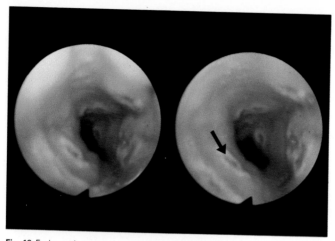

Fig. 18 Endoscopic appearances of HSV oesophagitis.

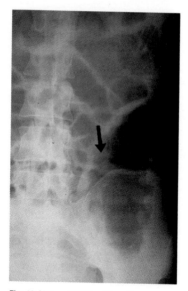

Fig. 19 X-ray of CMV colitis with 'thumbprinting' and thickening of bowel wall due to oedema.

	Cryptosporidiosis
Pathology	Infection with the protozoan, *Cryptosporidium parvum* causes mild symptoms in the immunocompetent, but in AIDS it persists and can be progressively fatal. It affects any portion of the GIT, particularly the small bowel and biliary tree (10%). Most patients will be profoundly immunocompromised (CD4 count $< 100 \times 10^6/l$).
Clinical features	Severe watery diarrhoea and anorexia are usual. Vomiting and nausea characterize biliary involvement. Episodes last for weeks or months.
Diagnosis	Ziehl–Neelson staining demonstrates cysts of *C. parvum* in stool specimens (Fig. 20).
Management	Oral rehydration solutions and nutritional supplements are useful and symptomatic relief should be attempted. Many cases improve when anti-retroviral therapy is commenced.

	Mycobacterial infection
Pathology	*Mycobacterium avium intracellulare* complex affects the GIT in severely compromised patients. Acid-fast organisms are found in stools or biopsies (Fig. 21).
Clinical features	Fever, night sweats, periumbilical pain and diarrhoea.
Management	A combination of anti-mycobacterial drugs, including clarithromycin and rifabutin, and anti-retroviral agents.

Other gastrointestinal infections

Infection with *Salmonella*, *Campylobacter* and *Shigella* is probably no more common or severe than in the general population. However, in patients with a low CD4 cell count, there is a higher propensity for salmonella infection to become bacteraemic. Recurrent salmonella bacteraemia is an AIDS-defining event. Suitable specific therapy is with a quinolone antibiotic such as ciprofloxacin for 2 weeks. Diagnosis is confirmed by stool and blood culture.

Protozoa other than cryptosporidia can also cause diarrhoea, including the microsporidia (*E. bieneusi* and *E. septata*) and *Isospora belli*. These organisms may respond to anti-microbials linked to anti-retroviral therapy.

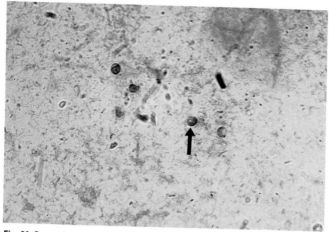

Fig. 20 Cysts of *Cryptosporidium parvum* in stool specimen.

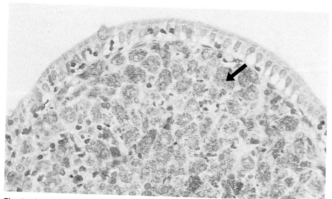

Fig. 21 Small intestinal biopsy showing lamina propria histiocytes and numerous atypical AAFBs.

Problems affecting the entire gastrointestinal tract

Kaposi's sarcoma (see also Chs 9, 10 & 15)

Clinical features

Visceral or intestinal Kaposi's sarcoma (KS) is usually asymptomatic but may give rise to perforation, obstruction or haemorrhage. Jaundice may result from biliary obstruction. Protein-losing enteropathy due to mesenteric lymphatic obstruction is described.

Diagnosis

Filling defects occur on barium studies (Fig. 22). Flat or polypoid, purple lesions are seen on endoscopy (Fig. 23). Biopsy features are similar to those of KS elsewhere.

Management

KS frequently resolves when the immune system improves following highly active anti-retroviral therapy. In persistent cases cytotoxic chemotherapy may be required.

Lymphoma (see also Chs 7, 9, 10 & 15)

Clinical features

The GIT is the commonest site for extranodal lymphoma in AIDS. Presentation depends on the site:
- Dysphagia and chest pain in oesophagus
- Haematemesis in gastric disease (Fig. 24)
- Obstruction, perforation or intussusception (Fig. 25) with bowel tumours
- Altered bowel habit and bleeding with rectal lesions
- Hepatic and nodal masses are often asymptomatic.

Fever and night sweats are non-specific features.

Diagnosis

Localization with various imaging techniques must be followed by histological confirmation. Fine-needle biopsy, ascitic aspiration, peritoneoscopy or laparotomy all play a role.

Prognosis

Since the advent of highly active anti-retroviral therapy the prognosis of lymphoma has greatly improved with long-term remissions and possible cures. However, lymphoma is becoming more common.

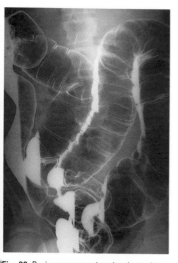

Fig. 22 Barium enema showing irregular mucosa and some narrowing of the sigmoid and rectum: KS.

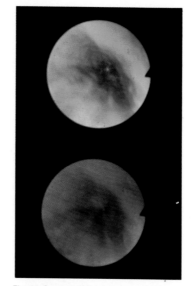

Fig. 23 Scattered bluish lesions of the duodenum consistent with Kaposi's sarcoma.

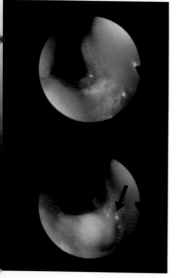

Fig. 24 Endoscopic appearances of ulcerated gastric lymphoma.

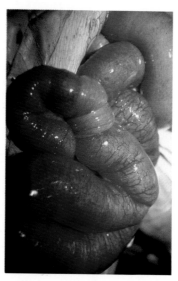

Fig. 25 Operative picture demonstrating ileal intussusception due to lymphoma.

Peri-anal disease

Anogenital warts

Aetiology
Ano-genital warts are caused by infection of the epidermis by human papilloma virus (HPV), which is usually sexually transmitted.

Pathology
Ano-genital warts are pleomorphic. Exophytic warts (condylomata acuminata) are commonest, but papular or flat forms and the common wart (verruca vulgaris) may occur. There is an epidemiological association between women with cytological evidence of HPV and cervical dysplasia. It is probable that this association is greater in the presence of HIV disease.

Clinical features
The commonest sites are the subpreputial area in men (Fig. 26) and the fourchette in women (Fig. 27). They also occur commonly in the urethral meatus, perineum, in the anal canal (Fig. 27) and on the vagina and cervix. Warts may also occur at extragenital sites, such as the mouth and the nipple. Genital warts tend to be more extensive and resistant to therapy in HIV infection.

Management
There are three main modalities of treatment:
- *Cytotoxic caustic agents* such as podophyllin, 5-fluorouracil and topical trichloroacetic acid (TCAA).
- *Mechanical surgery*, ablation by cryotherapy, electrocautery, diathermy, or laser.
- *Immune-modulating agents* such as Imiquimod cream.

Of these, podophyllin and cryotherapy are most commonly used, but intra-anal warts often require excision (Fig. 26).

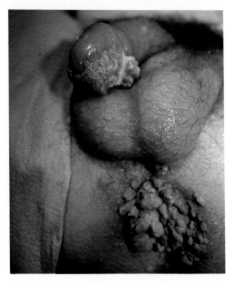

Fig. 26 Anal and penile condylomata prior to surgical excision.

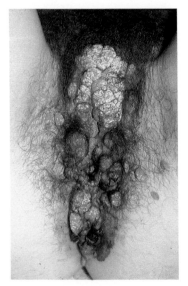

Fig. 27 Anogenital warts involving perineum and extending into anal and vaginal canals.

Peri-anal ulceration

This may be due to herpes simplex (Fig. 28), cytomegalovirus, severe candidiasis or very rarely, syphilis. Culture of swabs in viral or fungal media will usually establish the diagnosis with dark-ground microscopy and serology testing if syphilis is suspected. Biopsy may also be required.

Peri-anal tumours

Kaposi's sarcoma and anal carcinoma are more common in HIV-infected patients. Syphilitic condylomata should also be suspected.

Liver and spleen

Hepatosplenomegaly

The spleen is frequently enlarged in uncomplicated HIV infection. It may also be involved in lymphoma of both the non-Hodgkin's and Hodgkin's types. Liver enlargement is usually indicative of a problem complicating HIV such as lymphoma.

Hepatitis/jaundice

Acute and/or chronic hepatitis may be caused by the hepatotropic viruses A (acute only), B, C and D. These agents share many of the same routes of infection as HIV and hepatitis C is more severe in HIV-infected patients. Drugs, such as the protease inhibitors and anti-mycobacterial agents, can also cause hepatic inflammation. Cholestatic jaundice may be drug induced or caused by cholangiopathies related to infection with *Cryptosporidium parvum*, cytomegalovirus or direct HIV damage.

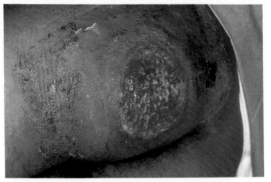

Fig. 28 Giant herpetic ulcer, from which HSV I was cultured. The lesion responded to acyclovir.

Conditions of the external ear, middle ear and inner ear can be manifestations of HIV infection. All of the conditions described in this chapter are now less commonly seen in the HAART era as in general they are associated with moderate to severe immunosuppression. However, these conditions may present in individuals who have undiagnosed HIV or are failing or have failed HAART.

External ear

The external ear suffers from many of the cutaneous conditions common elsewhere in HIV infection. Thus, seborrhoeic dermatitis, molluscum contagiosum, papillomata (Fig. 29) and KS are all common in this site.

Otitis externa

Aetiology

This may be idiopathic or secondary to otitis media, dermatitis or obstruction, e.g. by KS.

Pathology

Common infecting organisms are *Pseudomonas aeruginosa* and *proteus*. However, fungal infections such as *Aspergillus* do occur and can be very aggressive. *Pneumocystis carinii* has also been a reported cause.

Clinical features

Symptoms. Pain, discharge and deafness.

Signs. Otoscopy reveals a cream-coloured discharge usually obscuring the tympanic membrane (Fig. 30). An underlying cause, such as tumour or dermatitis, may be observed. Bacterial infection may spread causing cellulitis of the adjacent pinna.

Management

It is essential to send swabs for bacteriological and fungal microscopy and culture. Treatment should begin with aural toilet, aminoglycoside ear drops and analgesia. If cellulitis intervenes, i.v. benzyl penicillin and flucloxacillin are indicated. Any underlying cause should then be managed appropriately: dermatitis with topical steroids, and KS with the Argon laser.

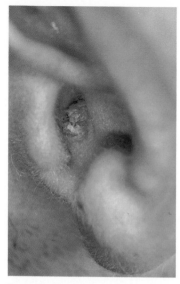

Fig. 29 These papillomata of the external ear were successfully treated by cryotherapy.

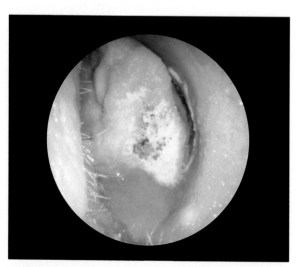

Fig. 30 Yellow exudate in otitis externa with black spores of *Aspergillus niger* visible.

Middle ear

Otitis media

Aetiology
This may be a primary infection, or there may be a preexisting condition such as perforation. Eustachian tube dysfunction secondary to benign follicular hypertrophy of the adenoids (Fig. 31), nasopharyngeal tumour, or upper respiratory tract infection has led to an increase in serous otitis media (glue ear; Fig. 32) in HIV infection.

Pathology
The effusion of serous otitis media contains few bacilli, but the HIV has been cultured within it. *S. pneumoniae, H. influenzae, Pneumocystis carinii* and *Cryptococcus neoformans* have been found in acute infections.

Clinical features
Serous otitis media presents with conductive deafness, and there may be a mass of adenoidal tissue in the postnasal space.

Acute otitis media presents with acute pain, deafness and unsteadiness. There is a red eardrum on otoscopy. Otorrhoea may ensue.

Management
Serous otitis requires ephedrine nosedrops 1%, and attention to underlying pathology: adenoidal blockage may be so marked as to require curettage for relief of symptoms and to exclude lymphoma. Failure of the effusion to resolve may require grommet insertion. In acute otitis media, oral amoxycillin and analgesia are prescribed. Failure to resolve in 48 h necessitates myringotomy and drainage, remembering to send pus for culture.

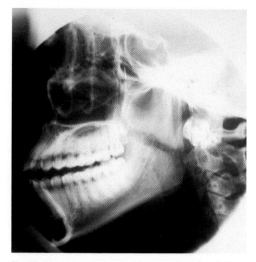

Fig. 31 Adenoidal enlargement shown on lateral neck X-ray.

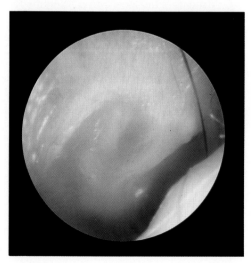

Fig. 32 Dull tympanic membrane in serous otitis media associated with adenoidal enlargement.

Inner ear

Sensorineural deafness

Aetiology

This has many potential causes: infections such as syphilis, cryptococcosis and toxoplasmosis, ototoxic medications, especially aminoglycosides and cytotoxics, and cerebral tumours. It is possible that primary HIV deafness occurs as part of generalized encephalopathy.

Investigations

These should include syphilis and toxoplasma serology and viral titres. Pure tone audiometry may show high-frequency loss (Fig. 33), and brainstem evoked responses may help to localize a lesion. If there is no obvious cause, an MRI scan is indicated.

Management

The underlying cause should be treated, but despite this, most cases do not improve and an hearing aid may be required.

Herpes zoster oticus

A common site of herpes zoster infection in HIV patients is the inner ear, causing the Ramsay–Hunt syndrome.

Clinical features

There is acute onset of severe pain with vertigo, deafness and a lower motor neurone facial palsy of variable severity. This is followed 24–48 hours later by a rash, often multidermatomal (Fig. 64, p. 66), and otoscopy may reveal vesicles (Fig. 34).

Management

Prostration may require i.v. fluids, vestibular sedatives and strong analgesia. Acyclovir should be commenced as soon as vesicles appear.

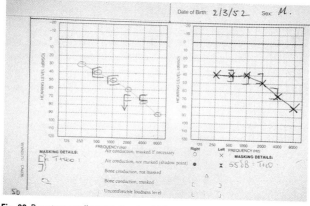

Fig. 33 Pure-tone audiogram showing high-tone sensorineural hearing loss.

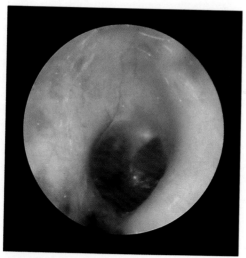

Fig. 34 Segmental vesiculation postero-inferiorly on otoscopy in Ramsay–Hunt syndrome.

Nose and sinuses

Chronic rhinosinusitis

This is very common in HIV infection, and may have an allergic basis. Candidiasis also occurs here.

Clinical features

These include rhinorrhoea, which may be purulent, and nasal obstruction of variable severity.

Management

Rhinoscopy, preferably with a flexible nasendoscope, is used to exclude obstructive lesions, e.g. KS and lymphoma. Swabs are taken for bacterial and fungal culture. Oral imidazoles, e.g. fluconazole are used to treat candidiasis, otherwise empirical treatment is with steroid sprays.

Acute sinusitis

Pathology

There is most often a mixed aerobic and anaerobic infection. Patients with AIDS may also harbour fungi, mycobacteria and *Legionella*, and the sinuses may act as a reservoir of such infections.

Clinical features

Acute pain and tenderness occurs around the cheek and orbit, with periorbital oedema (Fig. 35). Sinus X-ray may show a fluid level or opacity (Fig. 36).

Management

An antral washout provides symptomatic relief. The aspirate should be sent for culture. A broad-spectrum antibiotic and anti-fungal agent should be used, preferably intravenously.

External nose

This is a common site for KS (Fig. 37).

Mouth

Careful examination of the mouth in an immunocompromised HIV-infected patient may reveal lesions characteristic of HIV infection, e.g. oral hairy leukoplakia (OHL), bacterial fungal or viral infections, malignancy, e.g. KS, or clinical evidence of other systemic conditions associated with HIV, e.g. thrombocytopenia.

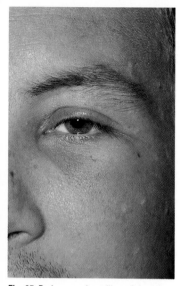

Fig. 35 Redness and swelling of the left cheek in acute sinusitis in an AIDS patient.

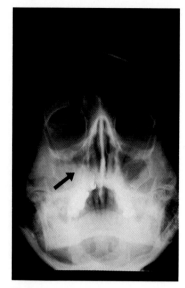

Fig. 36 Fluid level in left maxillary antrum is visible on this sinus X-ray of the same patient.

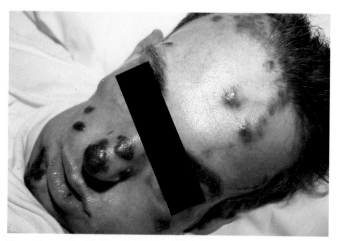

Fig. 37 Gross nodular Kaposi's sarcoma of the external nose. The submandibular gland is also involved.

Viral infections

Oral hairy leukoplakia

Oral hairy leukoplakia (OHL) has been regarded for some time as pathognomonic for HIV infection. Although occcasionally seen in immunocompromised transplant recipients, it is only since the advent of HIV that the condition has been characterized.

Pathology

It represents an opportunistic infection by the Epstein–Barr virus (EBV) within the mucosa of the oral cavity. Histologically it is characterized by epithelial hyperkeratosis with balloon cells and keratin hairs, and a lack of inflammatory response in 86% of cases (Fig. 38). By special staining, the virus can be visualized in various stages of replication within the epithelium (Fig. 39). The characteristic location of OHL on the tongue may be due to secretions of EBV by the salivary glands.

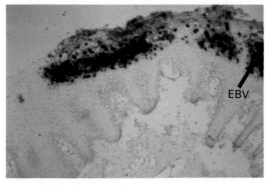

Fig. 38 Section of OHL showing hyperkeratosis keratin hairs. Balloon cells not clearly shown. In situ hybridization shows EBV.

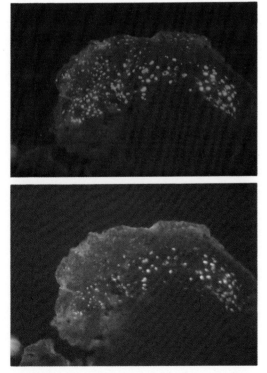

Fig. 39 Radioimmunofluorescent images: early antigen (green) and viral capsid antigen (red).

Clinical features	*Symptoms.* OHL is usually asymptomatic. Any discomfort is often due to the presence of an intercurrent candidal or other infection. It may spontaneously regress and relapse.
	Signs. Early OHL appears as isolated, often unilateral whitish patches on the sides of the tongue (Fig. 40). Later, it may become raised, corrugated, shaggy or remain flat. The commonest site is the lateral border of the tongue, but the dorsum of the tongue (Fig. 41), the floor of the mouth (Fig. 42), the cheeks and palate are all variably affected. In the most severe cases, OHL may take on a yellow or brownish appearance due to the drying of keratin (Fig. 41).
Differential diagnosis	OHL needs to be differentiated from oral candida with which it is often associated (see p. 51). Leukoplakia in sites atypical for OHL may represent dysplasia or neoplasia and thus warrant biopsy.
Management	The majority of cases require no specific treatment and regress with HAART. If discomfort is present, it should be treated as oral candidiasis.

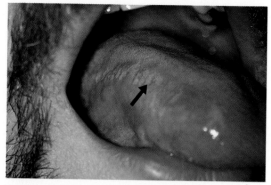

Fig. 40 A patient with early OHL affecting right side of tongue. Note also aphthous ulcers.

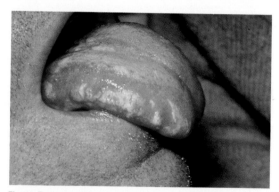

Fig. 41 Extensive OHL on sides and dorsum of tongue.

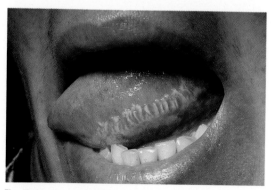

Fig. 42 A patient with AIDS: typical corrugations blend with flat OHL on the floor of the mouth.

Oral candidiasis

The association of oral candidiasis with AIDS was noted in the early 1980s. The appearance of oral candidiasis is variable.

Clinical features

The commonest appearance is the pseudomembranous form: a creamy plaque that may be wiped off to leave a bleeding surface (Fig. 43). Erythematous, or atrophic, candidiasis appears as red patches (Fig. 44), whilst leukoplakic candidiasis is white and firm and cannot be wiped off (Fig. 45). Angular cheilitis is a common perioral manifestation.

Differential diagnosis

Candidiasis must be differentiated from the various forms of leukoplakia, especially OHL (see p. 47). Unlike leukoplakia, scraping with a tongue depressor will remove candida in most cases. Where scrapings are possible, the finding of hyphae on microscopy will confirm a diagnosis of candida. In an older patient, leukoplakia may represent dysplasia and a biopsy would be indicated.

Management

Treatment is generally with oral imidazoles, e.g. fluconazole or with topical agents, e.g. nystatin mouthwashes or amphotericin lozenges.

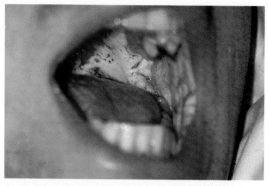

Fig. 43 Gross pseudomembranous candidiasis of oral cavity.

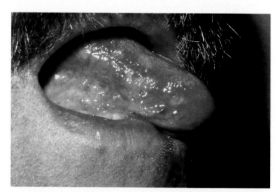

Fig. 44 Painful, red tongue in atrophic candidiasis.

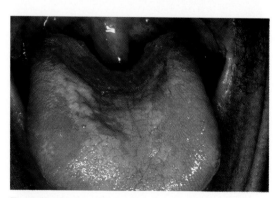

Fig. 45 Mixed leukoplakic and atrophic candidiasis in a patient with AIDS.

Viral infections

Herpes simplex (HSV)

Clinical features
Generally, this is self-limiting with restricted areas of vesiculation and ulceration healing in 7–10 days. With immunosuppression, this may become more generalized especially in perioral (Figs 46 & 47) and palatal (Fig. 48) regions, requiring oral acyclovir.

Other viruses

Clinical features
Cytomegalovirus (CMV) may cause ulceration clinically indistinguishable from aphthous ulceration (Fig. 52), whilst the warty condylomata acuminata of human papilloma virus have also been observed. Herpes zoster rarely involves the mouth.

Management
Any oral lesion not responding to therapy should be considered for biopsy to establish the diagnosis by histology and culture, including viral culture. Treatment is targeted at the causative agent, however symptomatic measures such as chlorhexidine mouthwash as antisepsis and/or topical anti-inflammatory agents, for example benzydamine, may be helpful.

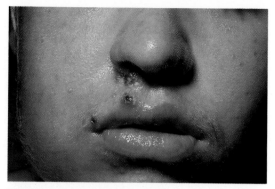

Fig. 46 Multiple perioral vesicles of HSV I.

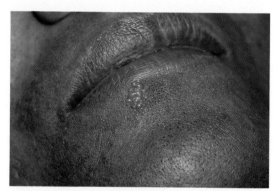

Fig. 47 Perioral vesicles producing HSV II on culture.

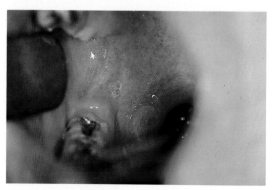

Fig. 48 Persistent, painful oral ulcer proving to be herpetic on biopsy. It responded to acyclovir.

Kaposi's sarcoma

This is a common site for presentation of Kaposi's sarcomata.

Clinical features

Early lesions are flat and bruise-like and are commonest on the palate (Fig. 49) and gingiva. However, they may become very large and ulcerated (Fig. 50). Symptoms are unusual, but large lesions may cause problems with deglutition or, rarely, airway obstruction.

Diagnosis

In the presence of other features of HIV infection and a characteristic appearance, biopsy is usually unnecessary, although it is sometimes required to rule out lymphoma or squamous cell carcinoma.

Management

Oral KS will generally recede with HAART. However if additional treatment is required, chemotherapy with vincristine and bleomycin is used. Local radiotherapy is effective but troublesome stomatitis is common.

Acute necrotizing ulcerative gingivitis (ANUG)

ANUG, or 'trench-mouth', is a bacterial infection which is now rare in the absence of malnutrition, but a similar condition is also seen in patients with HIV infection.

Clinical features

Bleeding, painful gums (Fig. 51) that may progress to ulceration and bony destruction.

Management

Topical povidone iodine and oral metronidazole are prescribed. Meticulous oral hygiene is necessary.

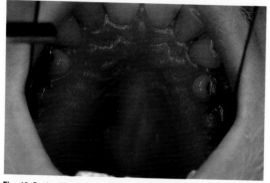

Fig. 49 Bruise-like patch of KS on hard palate.

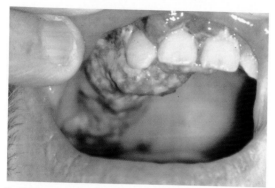

Fig. 50 Necrotic, ulcerating KS of upper jaw.

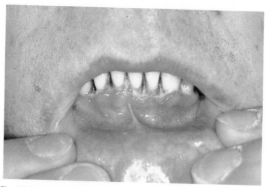

Fig. 51 Resolving ANUG with persisting necrosis of interdental papillae and no visible ulceration.

Aphthous ulceration

In HIV infection, these are common and tend to be recurrent and refractory to treatment.

Clinical features

Initially small white papules, which break down to form shallow ulcers. They may reach 1 cm or more in size (Fig. 52) and may occasionally become necrotic (Fig. 53), when diagnosis may be difficult. The commonest sites are the lips and buccal mucosa, rarely tongue and interdental locations. If extensive, aphthous ulcers may interfere with deglutition.

Differential diagnosis

Infectious lesions, especially herpes simplex and cytomegalovirus, and neoplastic lesions such as lymphoma or squamous cell carcinoma need to be excluded.

Management

Topical steroid preparations (Adcortyl in Orabase) facilitate healing, while lignocaine jelly gives some symptomatic relief. The most severe cases may be helped by the cautious use of thalidomide, taking care to stop if signs of neuropathy occur. Strong analgesia may be necessary for eating. If there is any doubt about the diagnosis, biopsy is mandatory.

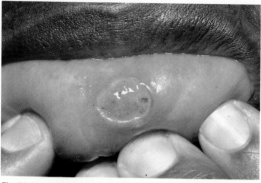

Fig. 52 Large aphthous ulcer of labial mucosa which responded to adcortyl treatment.

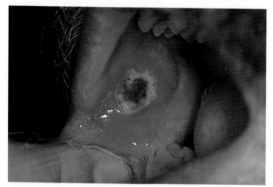

Fig. 53 Necrotic buccal aphthous ulcer.

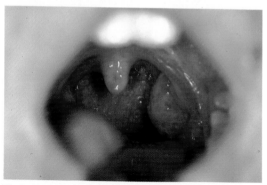

Fig. 54 This non-Hodgkin's lymphoma of the left tonsil was the presenting feature of AIDS in this man.

Lymphoma

Pathology

As with other AIDS lymphomas, these are non-Hodgkin's lymphomas and poorly differentiated. Some are associated with Epstein–Barr virus infection. Prognosis tends to be poor, although occasional idiosyncratic response to treatment does occur.

Clinical features

Lymphoma may present in the tonsil (Figs 54 & 55), alveolus, palate (Fig. 56) or cheek regions. They are painless unless infected but may rapidly ulcerate. It is essential to perform a full physical examination to exclude disseminated disease.

Diagnosis

A clinically suspicious lesion should undergo early biopsy, from which the histological features of lymphoma (Fig. 61, p. 64) are sought. A careful programme of investigation including chest X-ray, abdominal CT scan and bone-marrow biopsy is then undertaken to stage the disease.

Management

Localized lymphoma can be managed by radiotherapy, but the disease is usually widespread by the time of diagnosis. Hence, chemotherapy, e.g. vincristine and adriamycin, is generally required. HAART should be commenced.

Thrombocytopenia

Mild thrombocytopenia is particularly common in HIV infection. Symptomatic thrombocytopenia is now rare since this condition improves with HAART.

Clinical features

In the oral cavity, this presents as petechiae, ecchymosis (Fig. 57) or bleeding gums. Treatment is with platelet infusions in severe cases.

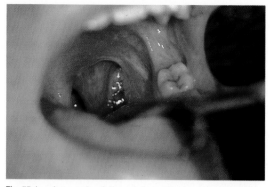

Fig. 55 Local regression followed chemotherapy, but intracranial spread caused death weeks later.

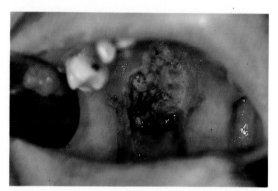

Fig. 56 This lymphoma presented as a necrotic ulcer of the hard palate.

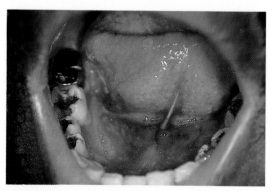

Fig. 57 Sublingual ecchymosis due to thrombocytopenia. Note also angular stomatitis and OHL.

Salivary glands

Parotid enlargement
This is a well-recognized presentation of paediatric AIDS (Fig. 142, p. 140), but also occurs in adult disease.

Pathology

The commonest condition is cystic enlargement, which may be due to sialadenitis (HIV may be cultured from saliva of infected patients) or may represent cystic degeneration of hyperplastic lymphoid tissue.

Clinical features

There is gradual, possibly massive, painless enlargement of the parotid gland (Fig. 58), which may be bilateral.

Differential diagnosis

The most important conditions to differentiate are intraparotid *Mycobacterium avium-intracellulare*, KS (Fig. 59) and lymphoma, although infections such as (MAI) may also involve salivary tissue.

Management

Fine-needle aspiration reduces the size of the mass, but may need to be repeated. It also provides material for cytology and culture. Neoplastic and infectious pathology should be managed as outlined elsewhere. Cystic change does not require specific treatment.

Xerostomia
Dryness of the mouth complicates 5–10% of AIDS cases. The aetiology is unknown, but chronic HIV sialadenitis probably plays a part. Specific treatment with synthetic saliva is occasionally required.

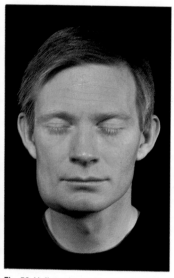

Fig. 58 Unilateral parotid enlargement in a 40-year-old man with AIDS.

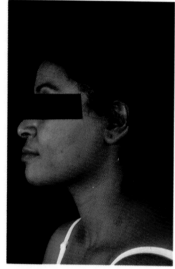

Fig. 59 Left parotid swelling due to KS.

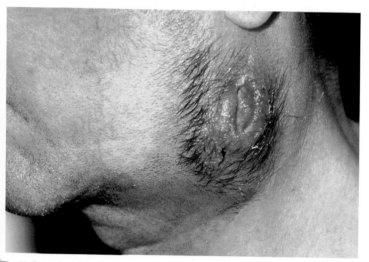

Fig. 60 Fungating wound 3 weeks after open biopsy of a neck mass. This proved to be lymphoma.

Cervical lymphadenopathy

The commonest cause in HIV infection is PGL (Table 1, p. 6), but the important differentials require description.

Differential diagnosis

Lymphoma. This is a common site for lymphoma to present. Unilateral, rapidly progressive nodal enlargement may be superimposed on PGL or occur 'de novo' (Figs 61 & 62). Constitutional symptoms, such as night sweats are common.

KS may spread to regional nodes.

Squamous cell carcinoma of the head and neck commonly metastasizes to cervical nodes. A primary site in the head and neck should be sought.

Mycobacterial infection. In AIDS, MAC is commoner than *M. tuberculosis*, and may occur even in the absence of chest disease (Fig. 121, p. 120).

Investigations

Full blood count may suggest infection, while skin tests may support a diagnosis of mycobacterial involvement. Fine-needle aspiration cytology is preferred to open biopsy of neck nodes, as only 10% of open biopsies uncover substantial pathology, and HIV patients heal poorly. Nevertheless, if suspicion of lymphoma remains, open biopsy becomes necessary (Fig. 60, p. 62).

Management

This depends on the underlying cause. Mycobacterial infections may recur.

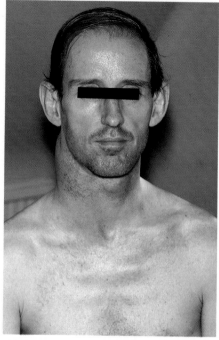

Fig. 61 Unilateral cervical lymphadenopathy: non-Hodgkin's lymphoma.

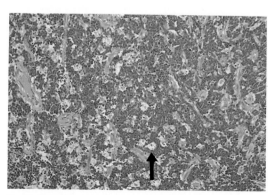

Fig. 62 'Starry sky' appearance of macrophages in AIDS-related non-Hodgkin's lymphoma. Reed-Sternberg cells not shown.

In the initial management of any patient with HIV infection, the skin and mucous membranes represent easily accessible areas to examine and biopsy. Patients may present with common skin infections which are more extensive or recurrent than usual, or with opportunistic infectious lesions from which a diagnosis of AIDS or HIV-related disease can be made. Many non-infectious skin problems are common.

Skin disorders due to infection

Herpes zoster

Clinical features
This is often multidermatomal (Fig. 63) and protracted. On healing, post-herpetic neuralgia or cosmetically damaging scarring may occur (Fig. 64).

Management
Given early, high-dose i.v. or oral acyclovir may limit spread. Famciclovir and penciclovir are also effective. Adequate analgesia is essential.

Wart virus

Clinical features
Wart virus infection, including the sexually acquired form, is very common in HIV infection. Verrucous lesions may be unusually extensive, or occur in unusual sites (Fig. 29, p. 40). There is rarely any doubt about the diagnosis (Fig. 90, p. 92).

Management
Topical treatment with keratolytics or cryotherapy is useful for cosmetically disabling lesions.

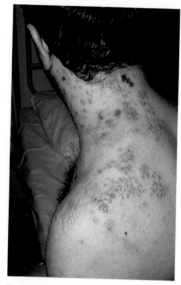

Fig. 63 Extensive herpes zoster affecting dermatomes C2–C4.

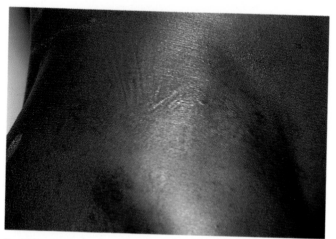

Fig. 64 Hypertrophic scarring and depigmentation following herpes zoster in AIDS.

Herpes simplex

Clinical features

In addition to the features described in Chapter 12, herpes simplex may give rise to giant or chronic skin lesions.

Management

Where diagnosis has been confirmed by viral culture or biopsy, acyclovir, penciclovir or famciclovir therapy is effective against chronic lesions.

Molluscum contagiosum

Aetiology

This represents infection with a pox virus, and occurs in up to 18% of patients with AIDS. It is spread by close physical contact.

Clinical features

Lesions are painless, pearly and umbilicated papules which may be very extensive (Fig. 65).

Management

If treatment is required for cosmetic purposes, cryotherapy or topical phenol may effect cure, but recurrence is common.

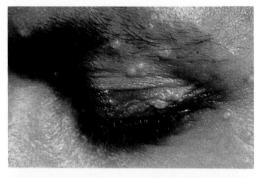

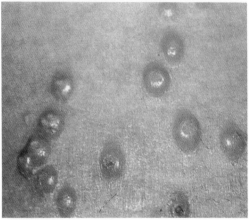

Fig. 65 Molluscum contagiosum affecting eyelid (above) and face (below).

Dermatophytoses

Clinical features

Cutaneous fungal infections are common and spread rapidly. Tinea pedis affects the feet, and *Trichophyton rubrum* affects the trunk and limbs. Onychomycosis, usually due to candidiasis, is common (Fig. 66).

Diagnosis

Hyphae may be demonstrated on potassium hydroxide preparation of scrapings or biopsies. Fungal culture may be necessary to select the best treatment.

Management

Topical therapy, e.g. with clotrimazole cream, should be tried, but unusually extensive or recurrent infections may require oral anti-fungals such as ketoconazole, fluconazole, itraconazole or terbinafine.

Other opportunistic skin infections

Clinical features

As part of disseminated opportunistic systemic infections, e.g. pneumocystosis, candidiasis, cryptococcosis or histoplasmosis (Fig. 67), skin lesions may occur. Where doubt exists, biopsy should be performed.

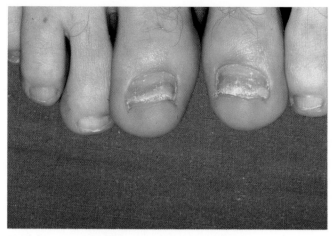

Fig. 66 Onychomycosis of feet.

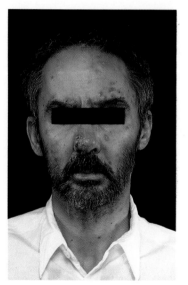

Fig. 67 Crusted facial papules in disseminated histoplasmosis.

Bacterial infection

Clinical features

In addition to staphylococcal infection (see p. 75), skin lesions may be associated with septicaemia, for instance due to *Salmonella* sp. Staphylococcal lesions may be unusually recurrent (Fig. 68).

Mycobacteria

Clinical features

Tuberculous lymphadenitis may break through the skin (e.g. 'collar-stud abscess'). In addition, there may be direct skin involvement producing violaceous lesions of lupus vulgaris (Fig. 69).

Mycobacterium avium-intracellulare (MAI), *M. kansasii* and *M. haemophilum* are sometimes also seen in this context.

Management

Appropriate anti-mycobacterial agents should be given as dictated by the species and sensitivity of the organism.

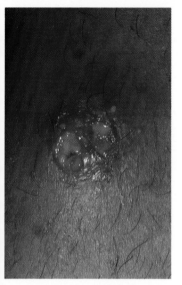

Fig. 68 Ecthyma in an AIDS patient.

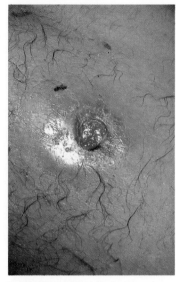

Fig. 69 Violaceous skin lesion, the culture of which produced mycobacteria.

Seborrhoeic dermatitis

This affects all groups of HIV-positive patients, and may be a presenting feature. About 80% of patients with AIDS are subject to the condition at some time during their illness.

Aetiology

This is unknown. Genetic predisposition is probably relevant, and infection with *Pityrosporum* species has been implicated.

Clinical features

Seborrhoeic dermatitis consists of a red, scaly rash most frequently affecting the cheeks, nasolabial folds, eyebrows and eyelids (Fig. 70). Thus, cosmetic disability can be great. The trunk and intertriginous areas may be involved (Fig. 71).

Management

Treatment is with topical steroid preparations, such as hydrocortisone, and anti-fungals, such as miconazole nitrate. Combination preparations of hydrocortisone and imidazole are useful. In resistant cases, systemic tetracycline or anti-fungals may be added. Once patients have been established on triple anti-retroviral therapy, the condition often improves.

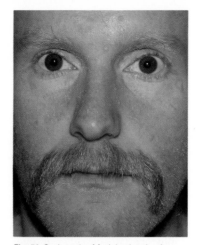

Fig. 70 Scaly rash of facial seborrhoeic dermatitis in a man with PCP.

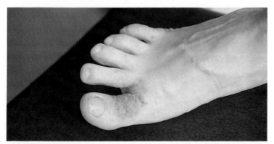

Fig. 71 Localized flaky plaque of seborrhoeic dermatitis.

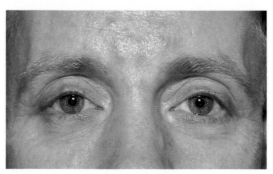

Fig. 72 Follicular blepharitis and acneiform folliculitis of forehead.

Folliculitis

Aetiology

In acute folliculitis, *Staphylococcus aureus* may be cultured. Biopsies of chronic lesions may show *Pityrosporum* yeasts within hair follicles. The cause of acneiform folliculitis is unclear, and culture of these lesions results in no growth.

Clinical features

Lesions consist of multiple slightly raised papules closely associated with hair follicles. They may occur on any hair-bearing site, though the upper trunk, neck (Fig. 73), limbs (Fig. 74) and intertriginous areas are most commonly affected. Acneiform folliculitis is characterized by a variety of particularly pruritic follicular lesions varying in distribution and degree (Fig. 72, p. 74, and Fig. 75).

Management

This condition may respond to topical anti-fungals with hydrocortisone, oral anti-fungals or anti-staphylococcal antibiotics. It often improves once anti-retroviral therapy is instituted.

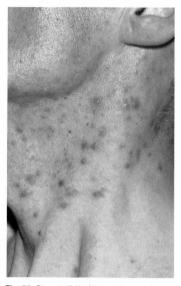

Fig. 73 Chronic folliculitis of face and neck.

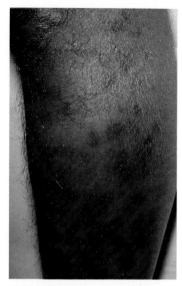

Fig. 74 Folliculitis of leg in a patient who was also a nasal carrier of *S. aureus.*

Fig. 75 Some of these acneiform folliculitis lesions have been scratched due to pruritus.

Kaposi's sarcoma (KS)

Until the advent of AIDS, the tumour first described by Moritz Kaposi in 1872 remained rare. Until the advent of potent anti-retroviral therapy, it was one of the commonest index conditions of AIDS and its recognition has attained considerable importance.

Incidence

In untreated patients, this varies depending on the risk group considered:
- *Homosexual men* 21%
- *Transfusion recipients and i.v. drug users* 3–4%
- *Haemophiliacs* less than 1%.

The incidence in homosexual AIDS cases appears to be declining.

Aetiology

KS is associated with cellular immunodeficiency. There is now considerable evidence that it is related to infection with a herpes virus (KSHV/HHV8). In addition, genetic predisposition (e.g. HLA-DR3) and male gender play a part.

Pathology

Histologically, KS consists of collections of endothelial-lined spaces separated by proliferating spindle cells (Fig. 76). The condition is invariably multifocal (Fig. 77). ➡

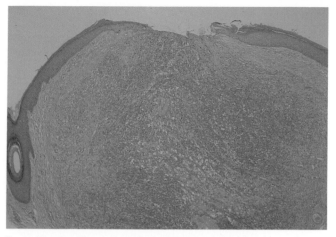

Fig. 76 Ulcerated KS and vascularized spindle cell proliferation.

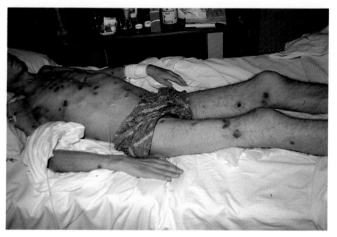

Fig. 77 Disseminated KS of trunk and limbs.

Clinical features

KS may occur in the later stages of HIV infection, and therefore is often concurrent with opportunistic infections and other features of AIDS. Early lesions (patch stage) are quite innocuous in appearance and somewhat resemble bruises (Fig. 78). Plaque stage lesions are less diffuse and slightly raised (Fig. 79). Later, lesions become nodular (Fig. 80) and may ulcerate. In colour, KS varies from pale pink, through violet, to dark brown. Initially, the lower limb is favoured, but KS may occur on any cutaneous surface including mucous membranes (see p. 55). In general, lesions are painless and non-tender, but considerable cosmetic disability often results.

Prognosis

Although normally indolent, when KS disseminates to viscera (see p. 33), serious and life-threatening complications may result. Conversely, lesions may occasionally regress spontaneously. ➤

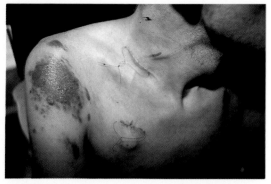

Fig. 78 Patch-stage lesion, showing bruise-like appearance.

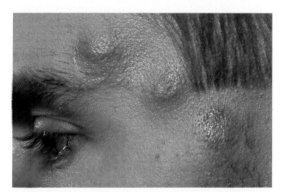

Fig. 79 Multiple, violaceous facial lesions of plaque-stage KS.

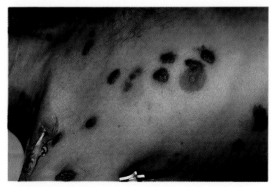

Fig. 80 Dark brown, nodular-stage lesions in advanced AIDS. Some are ulcerated.

Diagnosis	In a patient with known AIDS and classical skin lesions, biopsy is generally unnecessary. However, in view of the sometimes innocuous appearances of KS, all dermatological conditions in high-risk individuals need careful scrutiny and consideration for biopsy where doubt remains.
Management	A high proportion of KS lesions will regress once potent anti-retroviral therapy has been commenced and immunity starts to improve. Cutaneous lesions may be treated for cosmetic reasons with radiotherapy but may leave pigmented scars (Fig. 81). Extensive cutaneous lesions or visceral involvement may require the addition of cytotoxic chemotherapy, especially if resolution on anti-retrovirals is slow or the problems caused by KS are severe. Vincristine, bleomycin, doxorubicin or daunorubicin can be effective. Alpha-interferon is also useful in patients with high CD4 cell counts.
Complications	Lesions may ulcerate, and this may be severe (Fig. 82). KS may obstruct viscera, as described above. Lymphatic involvement is common, and lymphoedema may ensue (Fig. 83).

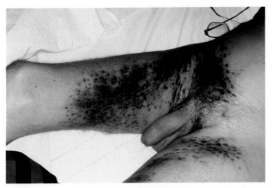

Fig. 81 Hyperpigmentation remaining after radiotherapy for KS of groin.

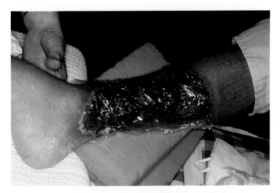

Fig. 82 Severe ulceration of advanced KS of lower limb.

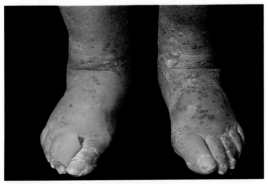

Fig. 83 Lymphoedema of legs following KS involvement of inguinal lymph nodes.

Scabies

Scabies can be atypical in presentation and cause a very extensive itchy, flaky rash ('Norwegian Scabies', Fig. 84) in patients with a low T-cell count. These patients are highly infectious as the lesions exude large numbers of mites and there have been several reports of outbreaks of scabies on wards and in clinics for HIV patients. Treatment with topical insecticides such as malathion repeated daily for 3 days can be effective but patients with high mite burdens may relapse. Ivermectin, an anti-protozoal agent has been reported to be effective in resistant cases.

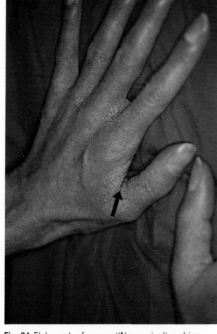

Fig. 84 Flaky rash of severe ('Norwegian') scabies.

Non-infective skin conditions

Vasculitis
Disseminated purpuric rashes are common. The aetiology is unknown.

Clinical features

Drug reactions
HIV-infected individuals are particularly liable to allergic reactions, which may take any form from red maculopapular eruptions (Fig. 85) to severe Stevens–Johnson-type reactions.

Psoriasis
This can be particularly severe with associated arthropathy and nail changes (Fig. 86). Management is the same as in HIV-negative patients, although may need to be more aggressive given the severity of psoriasis in many HIV-infected patients.

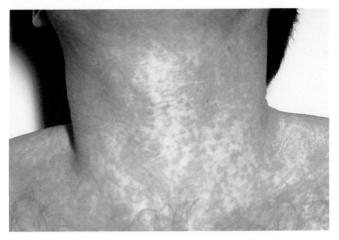

Fig. 85 Erythematous maculopapular reaction to septrin in a patient with AIDS.

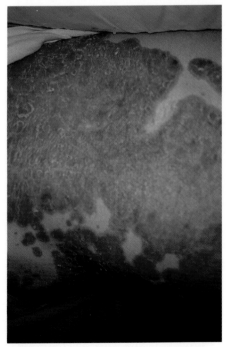

Fig. 86 Extensive truncal psoriasis in an HIV-positive man.

The onset of late disease is often heralded by non-specific features of fatigue, fever, abdominal pains and weight loss.

Fatigue and fever
Fatigue is a common manifestation of HIV disease. Patients may complain of being tired, particularly in the evening and after strenuous activity. If it is progressive or debilitating, it may represent worsening HIV disease or the presence of an opportunistic infection. Patients also frequently complain of fatigue in association with taking their anti-retroviral medication. 'Fever' may also be a non-specific symptom, although of course it can be associated with an opportunistic or other infection (see Ch. 7). Similarly non-specific night sweats are common and may or may not be associated with fever, but persistent or drenching night sweats could indicate an underlying opportunistic infection.

Joint and muscle pain
Reiter's syndrome has been reported in 6–10% of HIV-infected patients manifested by arthritis, urethritis, conjunctivitis and postular skin lesions. The major differential is psoriatic arthritis (see Ch. 16).

Weight loss
Progressive weight loss known as the HIV wasting syndrome (Fig. 87) or 'Slim disease' in Africa is a common manifestation of late-stage disease. It is defined by the CDC as an AIDS-defining illness when weight loss of more than 10% of body weight is associated with fever for more than 30 days or diarrhoea in a known HIV-infected patient (see Ch. 2). Weight loss may result from HIV disease alone or may indicate an underlying infection or malignancy. As with all of the other AIDS-defining illnesses, Slim disease is now seen less commonly in the developed world.

The management of the Wasting syndrome involves highly active anti-retroviral therapy, nutritional supplements, possibly the use of appetite stimulants or occasionally anabolic therapies.

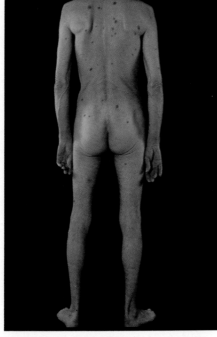

Fig. 87 Cachexia in HIV infection.

Patients with HIV infection should be offered screening for other sexually transmitted diseases (STDs) and contact tracing performed as appropriate. Genital ulceration in particular affects morbidity and the transmission of HIV (p. 7).

Genital herpes (HSV)

Pathology

Primary infection with HSV usually predates that with HIV. Both HSV I and II are seen. Acquisition is by contact of broken skin or mucous membranes with secretions or mucous membranes of a carrier (Fig. 88). The virus ascends via peripheral nerves, to establish latency within the ganglia.

Clinical features

Primary genital herpes is characterized by multiple, painful vesicles which may coalesce and ulcerate. Symptoms include dysuria, vaginal discharge due to cervicitis, and rectal discharge and tenesmus due to proctitis. Inguinal lymphadenopathy and systemic symptoms of fever, aches and pains may coexist. Episodes last about 2 weeks, but immunosuppression may prolong the episode or encourage dissemination.

Recurrent HSV presents as parasthesiae and pain, with vesicles and ulcers. In AIDS, recurrences increase in frequency and may last for weeks. Herpetic ulceration lasting more than 4 weeks is an AIDS-defining illness. Ulceration may be particularly severe, extensive and atypical (Fig. 89).

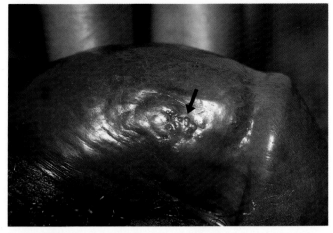

Fig. 88 HSV type I was cultured from this case of genital herpes in HIV infection.

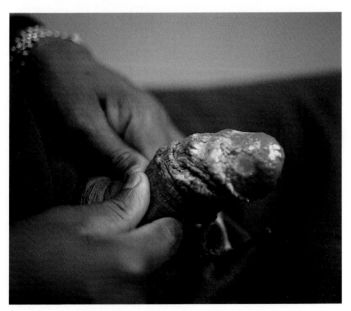

Fig. 89 Severe penile ulceration due to herpes simplex in a man with AIDS.

Primary disease. Confirmation is by viral culture of vesicle or ulcer fluid. Acyclovir, penciclovir and famciclovir are effective but may need to be in more prolonged courses (up to 10 d) in severe attacks.

Recurrent disease. Maintenance acyclovir therapy is recommended for all patients with HIV suffering recurrences.

Disseminated disease requires high-dose parenteral therapy. Foscarnet is an alternative in resistant cases.

Genital warts (see anogenital warts, Ch. 8)
Genital warts (Fig. 90) can be extensive and recur frequently in immunocompromised patients, although this situation may dramatically improve once a potent anti-retroviral regimen has been established.

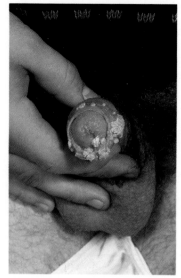

Fig. 90 Multiple warts of the penis.

Vulvovaginal and anorectal candidiasis

Aetiology

The causative agents are largely candida species such as *Candida albicans* and *C. krusei* but also other yeasts, especially *Torulopsis glabrata*. Many of these organisms are carried as commensals in the gut and on the skin. Clinical disease, including oral candidiasis, becomes more likely as the immune system declines in parallel with a fall in the CD4+ lymphocyte count.

Clinical features

Patients with vulvovaginal candidiasis present with pruritus and vaginal discharge. There may be local pain, external dysuria and superficial dyspareunia. On examination, there is vulval oedema with surrounding inflammation, vaginal mucosal erythema or superficial erosions. The discharge is classically likened to 'cottage-cheese' (Fig. 91), but it may also be thin, homogenous or scanty. The appearance of perianal disease is similar, with intertrigo possibly extending between the buttocks (Fig. 92).

Diagnosis

Vaginal symptoms due to *Trichomonas vaginalis* (TV) and bacterial vaginosis may be excluded by examining a direct smear from the posterior fornix under dark ground microscopy. Fungal hyphae may be visualized on a Gram's stain of vaginal discharge or by examining scrapings from intertriginous areas after potassium hydroxide application. The responsible organisms may be cultured on a suitable medium such as Sabouraud's and in non-responsive cases species identification and in vitro anti-fungal sensitivity performed.

Management

Most cases will respond to a topical imidazole such as clotrimazole, although occasionally the organism has inherent or acquired resistance to the topical agents and may require oral therapy with fluconazole, ketoconazole or itraconazole. In the past, patients with recurrent infection required long-term suppressive therapy with an oral agent, but this is usually not required if highly active anti-retroviral therapy (HAART) is used.

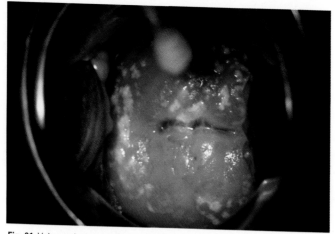

Fig. 91 Vulvovaginal candidiasis: white plaques of candida are adherent to the cervix.

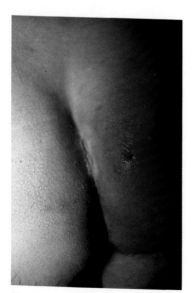

Fig. 92 Perianal intertrigo extending into natal cleft. There is also a buttock abscess.

Gonorrhoea

Incidence

Statistics for new cases of gonorrhoea dropped rapidly at the onset of the AIDS epidemic, but this was not sustained.

Clinical features

Gonorrhoea may be asymptomatic, especially in female patients. Urethral (Fig. 93), rectal, pharyngeal, cervical and disseminated gonorrhoea have been reported in HIV, with site-specific symptoms. Treatment is with an appropriate antibiotic such as ciprofloxacin.

Syphilis

This infection is still common in many developing countries and rises in incidence have been seen in recent years in the USA. It is less common in most developed countries including the UK. However, syphilis and other genital ulcerative (Fig. 94) diseases have been found to be important co-factors in the transmission of HIV. Patients with postprimary syphilis seem to be more susceptible to neurological disease and may be more resistant to therapy in the late stages of HIV disease.

Other STDs and anogenital problems

STDs sometimes seen include hepatitis B, chancroid, lymphogranuloma venereum and scabies. Kaposi's sarcoma (KS) is seen on genital skin and mucous membranes and may produce inguinal lymphadenopathy (Fig. 95). Male homosexuals with HIV infection are particularly prone to infected perianal conditions (Fig. 96).

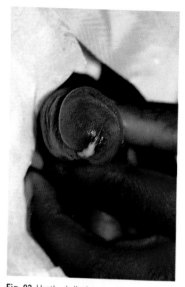

Fig. 93 Urethral discharge of gonococcal infection.

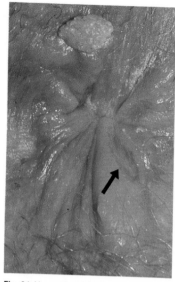

Fig. 94 Unusual multiple primary chancres of syphilis in the perianal area. Note also genital warts.

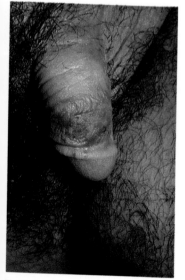

Fig. 95 Purplish patch of KS on penis.

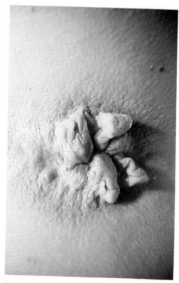

Fig. 96 Pruritic perianal skin tags in a man with HIV infection.

Neurologic complications of HIV are common and diverse. These complications may be due to a direct effect of HIV on the central nervous system or peripheral nervous system, an opportunistic infection or malignancy, particularly in the central nervous system. These complications may present as a space-occupying lesion or meningitis, or they may result as a side-effect of highly active anti-retroviral therapy (HAART).

Primary neurological disease

HIV encephalopathy (AIDS dementia complex)   The AIDS dementia complex syndrome is thought to relate pathologically to an effect of HIV-1 itself, but the association between the virus and the brain injury is not fully understood. Histologically, it can be divided into three subsets: 1) multi-nucleated giant cell encephalitis (Fig. 97); 2) loss of myelin staining; and 3) vacuolar myelopathy (Fig. 98).

Clinical features

Patients initially complain of difficulty in concentrating, forgetfulness, and trouble performing complex tasks or processing information. As the disease progresses, this poor concentration and forgetfulness gets worse and interferes with tasks of daily living. The patient will become more generally confused. Behavioural change may accompany this with loss of interest and apathy. AIDS dementia complex may be easily confused with depression. There are usually some subclinical motor abnormalities found on examination, e.g. hyper-reflexia, which can be helpful to diagnosis. In patients in whom vacuolar myelopathy is the underlying pathology, motor abnormalities are more marked, e.g. problems with walking associated with spasticity and ataxia.

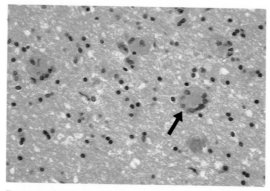

Fig. 97 Brain biopsy from a patient with subacute encephalitis showing characteristic giant cells.

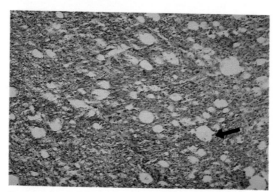

Fig. 98 Vacuolar myelopathy in a patient with lower limb weakness.

Psychological testing reveals cognitive defects of varying severity. CSF findings are non-specific but there may be mild elevation of protein, mild elevation in white cell count and elevated HIV viral load. However, none of these findings are specific. Computerized tomography (CT) and magnetic resonance imaging (MRI) scans are usually normal until the late stages when cortical atrophy becomes evident (Fig. 99).

HAART has greatly affected the incidence of HIV encephalopathy. In choosing anti-retroviral therapy, it is important to have one and preferably two drugs which cross the blood-brain barrier. For example, zidovudine, stavudine and Abacavir of the nucleoside reverse transcriptase inhibitors and Nevirapine a non-nucleoside reverse transcriptase inhibitor, have favourable central nervous system (CNS) penetration. However, the only protease inhibitor reported to penetrate the CSF appreciably is Indinavir.

Atypical aseptic meningitis

This can occur as part of the HIV seroconversion illness or during the period of transition from asymptomatic to symptomatic infection as the T-cell count drops to the range of 200/cmm or less. Clinical features are characterized by headache with variable focal signs – especially cranial nerve palsy – which tend to recur. Examination of the CSF usually shows pleocytosis and a raised protein level. Therapy is aimed at controlling symptoms and combined with HAART, as in HIV encephalopathy above.

Myelopathy

As mentioned above, patients may present with signs of long tract disease in the absence of any dementia-like symptoms representing involvement of the spinal cord by vacuolar myelopathy (Fig. 98). Again treatment is with HAART.

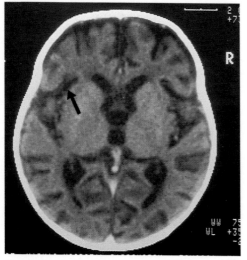

Fig. 99 CT scan of a patient with AIDS dementia syndrome with enlarged sulci of cortical atrophy.

Neuropathy

Clinical features

Cranial neuropathy.   Cranial nerve palsies may occur as part of atypical aseptic meningitis or HIV encephalopathy, e.g. Bell's Palsy (Fig. 100). However, these palsies may also be a presenting symptom of intracerebral space-occupying lesions secondary to opportunistic infections, e.g. toxoplasmosis or cerebral lymphoma.

Chronic polyneuropathy.   Both acute and chronic inflammatory demyelinating polyneuropathy have been described. These have an autoimmune aetiology in association with HIV. The commonest form is painful sensory neuropathy (Fig. 101). The acute inflammatory demyelinating neuropathy presents as a Guillian Barré-type syndrome. These patients usually respond to treatment with i.v. immunoglobulin, plasma exchange or corticosteroid therapy.

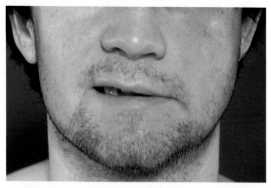

Fig. 100 Left facial weakness due to Bell's palsy in a man with stage IV disease.

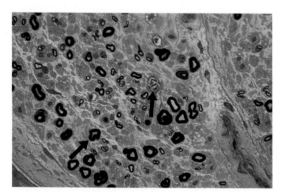

Fig. 101 Sural nerve biopsy in sensory neuropathy: decreased myelinated fibres, some degenerate.

Opportunistic infections of the CNS

Opportunistic infections of the CNS are common in AIDS or when the T-cell count is less than 200/cmm. However, these have now become much less common in the era of HAART. Pathologies presenting as space-occupying lesions include toxoplasmic encephalitis and primary cerebral lymphoma.

Toxoplasma gondii

Toxoplasmosis is one of the commonest of human infections, with seropositivity ranging from 20–70% in the USA. Infection is often subclinical in healthy individuals, but reactivation in HIV infection can be life threatening.

Pathology

Acute focal or diffuse meningoencephalitis with cellular necrosis associated with tachyzoites is seen (Figs 102 & 103). Necrotizing granulomas with little inflammation are characteristic. Thrombosis of blood vessels causing large areas of coagulation necrosis may produce mass lesions (Fig. 104).

Clinical features

Initial symptoms are headache and lethargy followed by focal signs. Untreated, seizures, confusion and impaired conscious level ensue. The condition may be fatal.

Investigations

Serological tests are unreliable, although toxoplasma antibody is usually present.

CT or MRI scans may reveal focal abnormality or may be normal. Where there is reasonable suspicion, empirical treatment should be instituted. Definitive diagnosis rests on brain biopsy.

Management

Six weeks of pyrimethamine and sulphadiazine are used, with indefinite maintenance therapy. Therapeutic response is usually monitored by repeating CT/MRI scans after 2 and 6 weeks of therapy. Although indefinite maintenance therapy is currently still used with immune reconstitution secondary to HAART discontinuing maintenance therapy can be considered when the CD4 counts remain greater than 200/cmm.

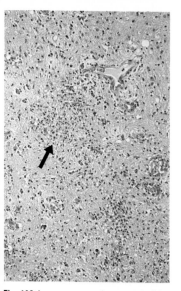

Fig. 102 Low power meningoencephalitis in cerebral toxoplasmosis pseudocyst and inflammatory response seen.

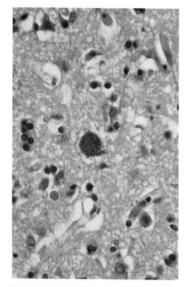

Fig. 103 Biopsy from a frontal lobe pseudocyst. High power, toxoplasma tachyzoite is seen centrally.

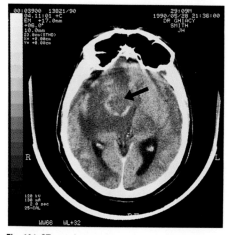

Fig. 104 CT scan in toxoplasmosis: ring-enhancing lesion with surrounding oedema and mass effect.

Primary cerebral lymphoma

Pathology

These are large cell lymphomas similar to those previously seen in other immunosuppressed states.

Clinical features

Presentation may be with encephalopathy, brainstem abnormality or cranial neuropathy. The CSF is often normal, but may contain elevated protein or atypical cells. CT or MRI scans demonstrate hypodense areas with peripheral enhancement (Fig. 105).

Differential diagnosis

Other space-occupying lesions, especially infections such as toxoplasmosis and other neoplasias. Where doubt exists, brain biopsy under stereotactic guidance is indicated.

Management

Radiotherapy and chemotherapy may slow the progress of primary cerebral lymphoma, however even in the era of HAART, the prognosis is expressed in months only.

Other tumours

Systemic lymphoma involving the CNS may occur, and especially affects the meninges, causing cranial neuropathy.

Kaposi's sarcoma may spread to the brain.

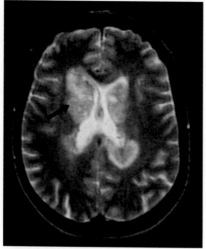

Fig. 105 MRI brain scan showing extensive periventricular areas of high signal intensity which proved to be lymphoma on biopsy.

Cryptococcus neoformans

Infection with this organism was the commonest fungal infection of the CNS; prior to HAART it complicated the course of AIDS in 5–15% of patients. Cryptococcol meningitis represents disseminated cryptococcol infection. The route of infection is via the respiratory tract and disseminated through the bloodstream into the CNS.

Clinical features

Patients with cryptococcal meningitis present with headache, sometimes associated with confusion, focal signs (Fig. 106) or seizures. CT and MRI scans are usually normal but may show cerebral atrophy or hydrocephalus or, rarely, an associated cryptococcoma (Fig. 107).

Investigations

India ink preparations (Fig. 108) of CSF give rapid diagnosis, then confirmed by culture. Latex agglutination for cryptococcal antigen is positive in meningitis.

Management

Therapy for cryptococcol meningitis is with i.v. amphotericin B and 5-fluocytisine. In mild cases the imidazole fluconazole can be used. Permanent maintenance therapy, usually with fluconazole is required, unless immune reconstitution with HAART occurs.

Other infections

Mycobacteria. MTB can cause both meningitis and tuberculoma in HIV infection.

Candida albicans can extend to the CNS, usually in cases of disseminated candidiasis.

Coccidiodomycosis is a persistent problem in HIV patients in the southwestern USA in particular. Most present with a chronic relapsing meningitis.

Bacteria are infrequently involved in infections of the CNS in HIV patients.

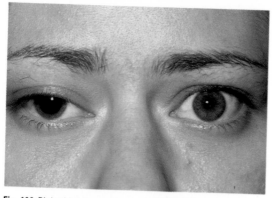

Fig. 106 Right third nerve palsy in a patient with cryptococcal meningitis.

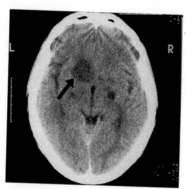

Fig. 107 *Cerebral cryptococcoma: low attenuation lesion initially treated as toxoplasma.*

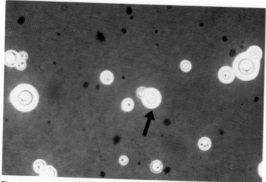

Fig. 108 *Cryptococcus neoformans* demonstrated by India ink preparation of CSF from an obtunded patient.

Progressive multifocal leukoencephalopathy (PML)

PML is an opportunistic infection of the brain caused by a human papova virus, called 'JC' virus. This infection usually occurs when the T-cell count is less than 200/cmm. It is a demyelinating condition, and hence can present with upper or lower motor neurone signs (Fig. 109).

Clinical features

The patient may progress with progressive mental aberrations or focal neurological deficits such as blindness, aphasia, or hemiparesis.

Pathology

Brain biopsy shows focal myelin loss with an absence of inflammation (Fig. 110).

Prognosis

Cytosine arabinoside has been reported to help. However, most cases progress slowly to death.

Treatment

Remission of PML can occur when patients have started HAART and this appears to correlate with a rise in CD4 T-lymphocyte count, which probably represents a restoration of the host immune response to JC virus.

Toxic peripheral neuropathies

Toxic sensory neuropathies may be difficult to distinguish from HIV-related distal sensory polyneuropathies. Toxic axonal neuropathy is caused by some of the anti-retroviral drugs, specifically zalzitabine (DDC), didanosine (DDI) and stavudine (D4T). In order to differentiate this neuropathy from HIV-associated neuropathy, a careful drug history must be taken. Remission following cessation of the suspected causal drug aids in diagnosis. Treatment is otherwise symptomatic by attempting to control pain.

CMV myelitis. CMV myelitis presents subacutely with bladder and/or bowel dysfunction and progressing leg weakness and sensory loss. It is treated with specific anti-CMV treatment such as ganciclovir after diagnosis is made by clinical suspicion and identification of CMV by PCR examination of the CSF. This disease occurs in the presence of low T-cell counts (normally < 50/cmm) and is rarely seen in the HAART era, except in untreated patients or patients failing therapy.

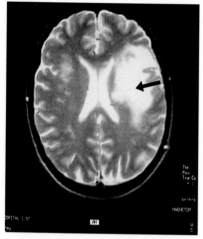

Fig. 109 MRI T2 weighted brain scan showing a large area of high signal intensity in the white matter of the left frontal and parietal lobes. There are smaller lesions in the remainder of the white matter. Of note there is no mass effect. These findings are consistent with PML.

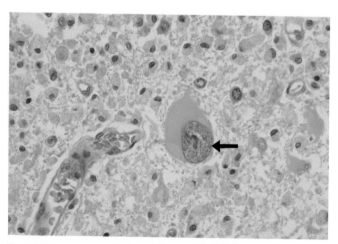

Fig. 110 High power magnification biopsy of frontal lobe in PML visible oligodendrocytes but astrocytes not seen indicating demyelination. Large viral inclusion body seen probably representing coincident CMV infection.

As many as 65% of AIDS patients are reported to have ocular pathology at some time, although this prevalence will inevitably fall as potent anti-retroviral drugs are used more. Of these, by far the commonest are cotton wool spots and CMV retinitis.

Cytomegalovirus (CMV) retinitis

Clinical features

Patients present with floaters or patchy visual loss, or may be diagnosed on routine screening. The involved eyes are not painful or red. There may be visual field defects with absolute scotomas. Fundoscopic findings are variable (Figs 111 & 112). CMV disease is normally only seen in patients with CD4+ lymphocyte counts of $<100 \times 10^6$.

Management

Ganciclovir, an inhibitor of viral DNA polymerase, is the treatment of choice. This is usually given i.v. for 2–4 weeks. Foscarnet and cidofavir are alternatives, the latter having the advantage of once weekly administration. In addition, these agents can be given by intravitreous injection. Once the disease has been controlled, prophylaxis is normally instituted in the form of oral ganciclovir, although alternatives include intravitreal injections or implants. Sometimes suppression with i.v. ganciclovir or foscarnet is required via an indwelling central venous catheter or cidofavir can be given bi-weekly via a peripheral vein. Many patients are able to stop suppressive therapy once they have been established on anti-retroviral therapy.

Prognosis

Untreated, progression to bilateral blindness within six months is usual. As these patients are profoundly immunosuppressed, they are at risk of early death from multisystem CMV disease or other AIDS-related problems unless they begin a potent anti-retroviral regimen. The prognosis has improved dramatically in recent years with improved HIV therapy.

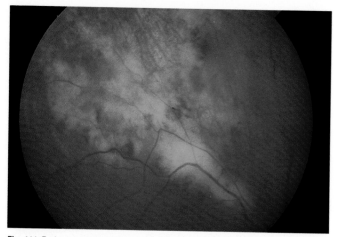

Fig. 111 Early, segmental CMV retinopathy showing areas of exudation and haemorrhage.

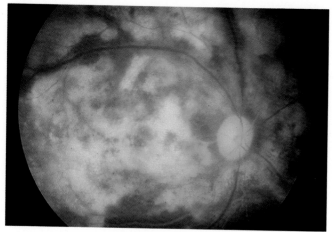

Fig. 112 Atrophic retina following CMV retinitis.

Other opportunistic ocular infections

Ocular toxoplasmosis, choroidal cryptococcosis, *Pneumocystis carinii* retinitis and choroidal mycobacterial granulomata have been described but are less common. Retinal haemorrhage may occur in zidovudine-related anaemia. It resolves with transfusion.

Cotton wool spots

Clinical features

These are superficial white retinal opacities that tend to spontaneously regress over a period of a few weeks (Fig. 113). They are thought to represent areas of ischaemia in the retinal nerve fibre layer and are not associated with any visual loss. Cotton wool spots tend to regress and recur during the course of HIV disease.

Differential diagnosis

Cotton wool spots may precede the development of overt CMV retinitis. It is therefore essential to perform serial observations. Other conditions causing cotton wool spots, such as diabetes, hypertension and collagen vascular disease are uncommonly found in HIV infection.

Conjunctival Kaposi's sarcoma

Clinical features

These may occur on any part of the conjunctiva, and are rarely large enough to cause visual disturbance (Fig. 114).

Differential diagnosis

Misdiagnosis of the lesions as haemorrhage or haemangioma is possible.

Management

If the lesions threaten vision or are cosmetically unacceptable, local excision or radiotherapy may be considered. This condition may spontaneously regress once triple anti-retroviral therapy is commenced.

Ocular motility disorders

Clinical features

Neuropathy/neuritis may affect cranial nerves III, IV or VI. In all cases, the possibility of intracranial pathology such as toxoplasmosis, cryptococcosis or lymphoma should be excluded (see Ch. 13).

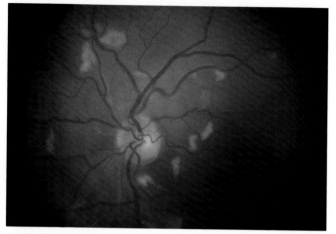

Fig. 113 Retinal cotton-wool spots.

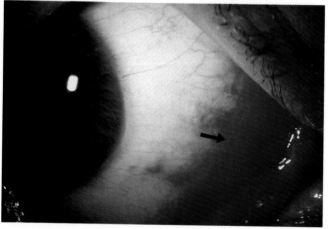

Fig. 114 Kaposi's sarcoma of right bulbar conjunctiva.

The cardiorespiratory manifestations of HIV infection have become less common in the era of HAART. The most common serious respiratory manifestation is pneumonia, which may be due to bacteria, mycobacteria or rarely viruses or fungi. Pleural effusions may also occur secondary to pneumonia but more commonly are secondary to malignancy such as Kaposi's sarcoma or lymphoma.

Pneumocystis carinii pneumonia (PCP) was the commonest index disease for AIDS in the pre-HAART era; 60% of AIDS patients developed PCP at some time. The introduction of prophylaxis against PCP prior to the introduction of HAART had already diminished the incidence of this opportunistic infection. Now PCP is seen most commonly in patients who are: (a) unaware of their HIV infection, (b) not adhering to their medication with HAART and/or PCP prophylaxis, or (c) failing HAART therapy.

Pneumocystis carinii pneumonia (PCP)

Pathology

Despite recent debate over taxonomy, *Pneumocystis* is probably best regarded as a fungus. Pneumonia appears to result from reactivation of infection that would be subclinical in the immunocompetent.

Clinical features

Initial symptoms are non-specific: anorexia and fatigue. These characteristically give way to a non-productive cough, low-grade fever and dyspnoea, which eventually occurs at rest. Symptom severity may be affected by the presence of PCP prophylaxis. Even with extensive disease, often the only chest signs are tachycardia and tachypnoea with normal breath sounds.

Investigations

Chest X-ray. Typical features are shown in Figure 115. Atypical features (Fig. 116) are not unusual, especially with prior PCP prophylaxis.

Arterial blood gases typically reveal hypoxaemia, but this may only be on exercise in mild cases. ➡

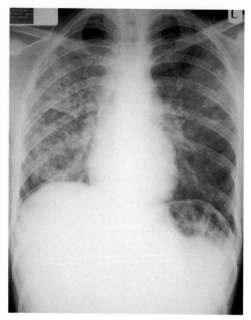

Fig. 115 Typical CXR of a moderately severe case of PCP: diffuse bilateral perihilar infiltrates.

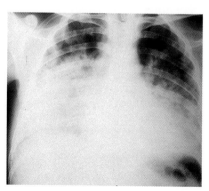

Fig. 116 Advanced PCP with widespread consolidation of mid and lower zones and some apical sparing.

Diagnosis	The diagnosis rests on identification of the organism histologically or by staining of samples of induced sputum or bronchoalveolar lavage (BAL) with immunofluorescent or silver stain (Figs 117–119).
Treatment	First-line therapy for PCP is trimethoprim (50 mg/kg/d) plus sulphamethoxazole (250 mg/kg/d) (co-trimoxazole), intravenously or orally for 21 days. Allergies to this drug are common (Fig. 86), and replacing with the equally effective sulphamethoxazole dapsone (100 mg/d) may be necessary. Clindamycin and primaquine can be given as an alternative therapy for patients who are unable to tolerate or who are allergic to either of the above regimes. In patients who fail to respond to any of the above treatments, salvage therapy with either i.v. pentamidine or methotrexate should be considered. Aerosolized pentamidine given once daily has been used to treat mild to moderate disease, when the patient is able to effectively receive therapy. Intravenous (i.v.) or i.m. pentamidine has also been used.
Prophylaxis	The CDC recommend prophylaxis for PCP in any HIV-positive patient whose CD4 lymphocyte count is less than 200 or 20% of total lymphocytes, or after the first attack of PCP. Several prophylactic regimens have been shown to be effective, including low-dose co-trimoxazole 5–7 times a week, nebulized pentamidine 300 mg 2–4 times a month, dapsone 100 mg and pyrimethamine 25 mg once or twice weekly. The choice depends on local resources, and the compliance and allergic profile of the individual patient. If following the commencement of HAART, patients maintain their T-cell counts >200/cmm, withdrawal of PCP prophylactic medication can be considered.

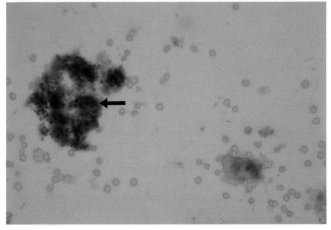

Fig. 117 Grocott's stain of a BAL specimen with pneumocysts staining blue-green.

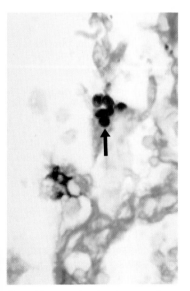

Fig. 118 Lung section showing cysts of *Pneumocystis carinii*.

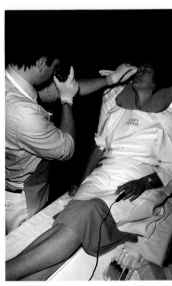

Fig. 119 Bronchoscopy in HIV-positive patient.

Mycobacterium tuberculosis (MTB)

Incidence

Tuberculosis is common in the HIV-infected population; it affects up to 14% of all patients with HIV in parts of sub-Saharan Africa and up to 2–10% of AIDS patients in the developed world. Tuberculosis, whether pulmonary or extrapulmonary is an AIDS-defining illness. Multi-drug resistant MTB has emerged in recent years as a particular problem associated with HIV infection.

Clinical features

Reactivation of infection is usual, and the clinical picture depends on the level of immunocompetence. In AIDS, the course tends to be more typical of progressive primary disease. Common presenting features are cough, fever, lymphadenitis (Fig. 120) and weight loss.

Diagnosis

Common radiographic findings are hilar or mediastinal adenopathy and lower or mid-lung field infiltrates. By contrast with non-HIV patients, apical infiltrates (Fig. 121) and cavitation are rare. Importantly, CXR may be entirely normal.

Examination of sputum and BAL for acid-fast bacilli is useful, and MTB may be subsequently cultured, even with a normal smear (50% of cases).

Management

Six months of anti-tuberculous therapy is the usual treatment course. Triple therapy is initiated usually with isoniazid rifampicin and pyrazinamide and reduced to two agents, usually rifampicin and isoniazid, after 2 months with the availability of culture and sensitivity. In patients in whom multi-drug resistance may be suspected, quadruple therapy by the addition of ethambutol to the above regime is prudent until sensitivity results are available. Prophylaxis against MTB is routine in some Centres, for patients who have positive tuberculin skin testing Heaf grade 3 or 4, although anergy is common in HIV infection. Some centres also recommend prophylaxis for all patients who are at high risk for MTB, e.g. immigrants from sub-Saharan Africa and i.v. drug users.

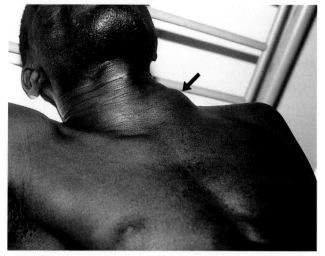

Fig. 120 There is a visible swelling in the left lower neck and supraclavicular area, which proved to be a tuberculous cold abscess.

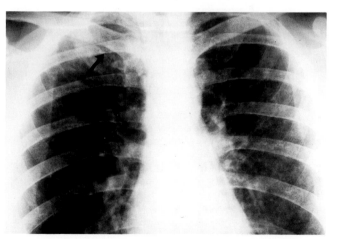

Fig. 121 Chest X-ray in tuberculous lung disease showing right apical infiltrates.

Atypical mycobacteria

Mycobacterium avium-intracellulare (*MAI*), *M. kansasii* and *M. xenopi* are often isolated from the lung in AIDS and may be incidental or part of disseminated disease.

Bacteria

Clinical features

Bacterial pneumonia is more common in patients who are immunocompromized with HIV infection than in the general population. The presentation is similar to bacterial pneumonia in the immunocompetent host with cough (usually productive), fever, dyspnoea and sometimes pleuritic chest pain. A range of organisms may be responsible, including common bacteria, e.g. *Streptococcus pneumoniae*, *Haemophilus influenzae*, (Fig. 122) or less common organisms, e.g. *Pseudomonas* species. Initial antibiotic therapy should be very broad spectrum (e.g. ceftazidime) until the cause is known.

Cytomegalovirus (CMV)

Pathology

CMV pneumonitis as a single pathology is unusual but it may cause a pneumonitis in patients whose T-cell count is less than 50/cmm. CMV is commonly isolated in BAL samples taken during the course of investigation for PCP. However the finding of CMV (usually by testing for CMV early antigen or seeing 'Owls-eye cells' on microscopy) may represent infection or simply may be due to colonization. Generally in this context, anti-CMV therapy is only initiated if the patient is slow to respond to anti-PCP treatment. Clinical features include progressive dyspnoea, dry cough and tachypnoea. Blood gas estimation will reveal hypoxaemia and chest X-ray will reveal interstitial infiltrates. Treatment is with the antiviral agents ganciclovir or foscarnet.

Clinical features

These include progressive dyspnoea and dry cough, with tachycardia, tachypnoea, hypoxaemia and interstitial infiltrates on CXR.

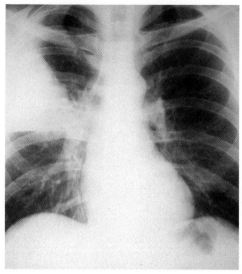

Fig. 122 Right mid-zone consolidation due to *H. influenzae,* which responded to penicillin.

Fungal infection

Cryptococcus neoformans can cause pneumonia, often as part of a disseminated infection. Histoplasmosis and coccidiomycosis also occur.

Clinical features

Signs of cryptococcal meningitis (p. 107) may be accompanied by cough, dyspnoea and haemoptysis. CXR shows well-defined nodules which may cavitate, or reticular shadowing (Fig. 123). Treatment is as for central nervous system involvement (p. 107).

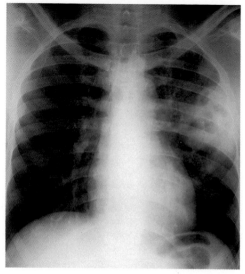

Fig. 123 Cryptococcal pneumonia: cavitating left mid-zone opacity consistent with fungal infection.

Kaposi's sarcoma (KS)

KS in the lung usually occurs as part of disseminated KS in the presence of severe immunosuppression. Prior to HAART, pulmonary KS was a common cause of death. However, KS often regresses in the presence of HAART and pulmonary involvement is now rarely seen in the developed world, although still common in sub-Saharan Africa.

Clinical features

KS may occur anywhere in the respiratory tract, causing obstruction, infection or haemorrhage. Dry cough, dyspnoea, wheeze and haemoptysis are seen. Respiratory failure may ensue.

Diagnosis

Nodular shadowing, pleural fluid and hilar adenopathy are seen on CXR (Fig. 124). Bronchoscopic visualization (Fig. 125) suffices for diagnosis if KS is present elsewhere.

Management

Radiotherapy or chemotherapy may be used for symptomatic cases.

Lymphoma

Unlike lymphoma in the general population, intrathoracic involvement is uncommon. However, it may give rise to pleural effusions, mediastinal adenopathy and recticulonodular infiltrates. Lymphoma is almost exclusively of the non-Hodgkin's B-cell type (Fig. 126).

Lymphocytic interstitial pneumonitis (LIP)

Originally described in children (see Ch. 18), this is now seen in adult AIDS, where some response to steroids has been reported in symptomatic cases.

Cardiac disease

HIV cardiomyopathy, HIV-related myocarditis secondary to opportunistic infection, e.g. with *Toxoplasma gondii* and pericarditis have all been described.

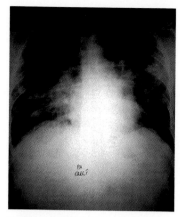

Fig. 124 Lung KS: right basal pleural effusion, coarse consolidation and some bilateral nodules.

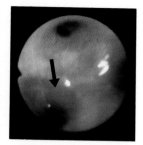

Fig. 125 Bronchoscopic view of submucosal KS in the trachea.

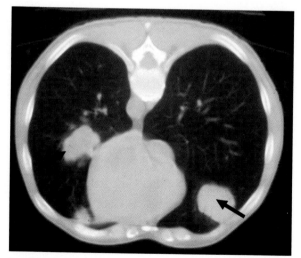

Fig. 126 CT scan in lymphoma with soft tissue lesions in both lung fields.

Reiter's syndrome

Incidence

This condition is reported to affect between 6 and 10% of HIV-infected patients at some time in their illness.

Clinical features

As in HIV-negative patients, it causes acute arthritis, usually of the larger joints (Fig. 127). It is often associated with sacroiliitis. Other symptoms of the classic syndrome are usually seen, including urethritis, conjunctivitis/iritis (Fig. 128), circinate balanitis (Fig. 129) and pustular/psoriaform rashes. A triggering infection is often found in either the urethra (chlamydia/NGU) or the gut, such as *Salmonella* or *Shigella*. The arthritis can be severe and chronic.

Management

Any triggering infection that is identified should be treated. The arthritis frequently requires therapy with intra-articular steroids in addition to non-steroidal anti-inflammatory drugs. Local or systemic steroid therapy may also be required for eye and skin complications. The prognosis in the era of active anti-retroviral therapy is unclear.

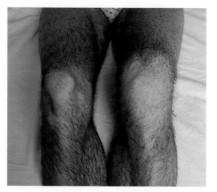

Fig. 127 Swollen left knee in a man with Reiter's syndrome.

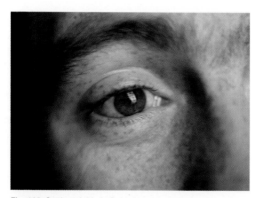

Fig. 128 Conjunctivitis in Reiter's syndrome.

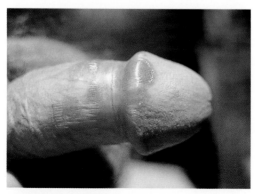

Fig. 129 Circinate balanitis.

Psoriatic arthritis (see Ch. 10)

Incidence

About 5% of HIV-positive patients have psoriasis of whom 10% will develop arthritis.

Clinical features

Arthritis is seen within the context of severe cutaneous psoriasis and is usually associated with nail changes (Figs 130 & 131). The pattern of joint involvement is similar to that in Reiter's syndrome. The arthritis usually takes a relapsing chronic course.

Management

Given that the psoriasis and arthritis can be severe, aggressive therapy may be required including systemic steroids or methotrexate. There have been reports of considerable improvement once potent anti-retroviral therapy has been commenced.

Myositis

Painful inflammatory myositis has been described in connection with HIV infection. This may be an autoimmune phenomenon, although viral inclusion bodies are sometimes seen on biopsy.

Myopathy

The commonest myopathy seen in AIDS is that related to zidovudine therapy (Figs 132 & 133). A condition similar to motor neurone disease has also been described. Painless myopathy related to mitochondrial dysfunction has also been reported.

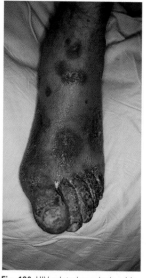

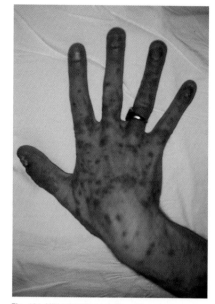

Fig. 130 HIV-related psoriasis with severe skin and nail changes and swelling of the Vth metatarso-phalyngeal joint.

Fig. 131 HIV-related psoriasis with severe dystrophy of the nails.

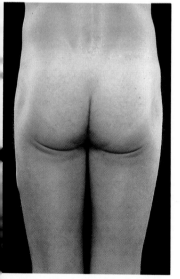

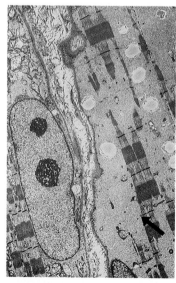

Fig. 132 Wasting of gluteal and quadriceps muscles in zidovudine-related proximal myopathy.

Fig. 133 Electron microscopy of muscle biopsy in the same patient showing atrophy of striated muscle fibres (arrow).

In addition to the sexually transmitted infections (Ch. 12) which affect the urogenital system, certain conditions have come to light that are specific either to HIV infection itself, e.g. HIV nephropathy and hypotestosteronism, or side-effects of anti-retroviral drugs, e.g. indinavir kidney stones.

HIV nephropathy

Different types of glomerulopathies have been described in HIV disease, the commonest however are focal and segmental glomerulosclerosis. It is commoner in blacks than in whites with a ratio of 3:1 and also in i.v. drug users. HIV-associated nephropathy can occur in both asymptomatic HIV infection and in AIDS, and with any T-cell count.

Clinical features

Patients usually present with proteinuria, often amounting to nephrotic syndrome and/or renal insufficiency. The onset is often abrupt and the progress rapid in the absence of treatment, with an interval from initial clinical presentation to dialysis of weeks to a few months. On abdominal ultrasound the kidneys are found to be enlarged. The diagnosis is now frequently made clinically, that is the presence of renal insufficiency, proteinuria (see Fig. 134) and enlarged kidneys in a patient who is HIV antibody positive. However, the diagnosis can be confirmed by identifying distinctive histological findings showing marked abnormalities in the glomeruli and tubular interstitium.

Treatment

Prior to the introduction of HAART, most patients with HIV nephropathy rapidly deteriorated and required dialysis. Zidovudine was the drug first shown to have an effect by producing temporary remission of the proteinuria, however disease progression with HAART appears to be halted. Other therapies which can be used are corticosteroids and angiotensin-converting enzyme (ACE) inhibitors. ACE inhibitors have been shown to improve renal insufficiency in HIV-associated glomulerosclerosis.

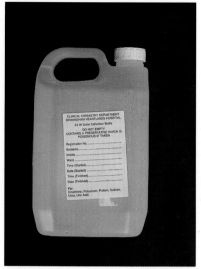

CLINICAL CHEMISTRY DEPARTMENT
BIRMINGHAM HEARTLANDS HOSPITAL

24 Hr Urine Collection Bottle

DO NOT EMPTY
CONTAINS A PRESERVATIVE WHICH IS
POISONOUS IF TAKEN

Registration No.

Surname

Initials

Ward

Time (Started)

Date (Started)

Time (Finished)

Date (Finished)

For:
Creatinine, Potassium, Protein, Sodium,
Urea, Uric Acid.

Fig. 134 24-hour urine collection bottle. In patients with proteinuria in HIV nephropathy, the quantity of protein loss in urine per 24 hours is measured.

Opportunistic infections and malignancies

In patients with advanced AIDS the kidney may be involved by CMV infection, extra pulmonary pneumocystis infection, mycobacterial infection and histoplasmosis in geographical areas where this is common. In cases of disseminated Kaposi's sarcoma and in non-Hodgkin's lymphoma, the kidney may be involved.

Hypotestosteronism and loss of libido

Loss of libido is a common complaint in men with advanced HIV infection. A significant proportion of men with asymptomatic HIV infection and a greater proportion of AIDS patients have been found to have low circulating free testosterone levels. The exact mechanism for this is unclear. The luteinizing hormone and follicle stimulating hormone may be normal or low and may respond to gonadotrophin-releasing hormone, thus suggesting that perhaps the low testosterone level is due to a disorder of the hypothalamus. It may be a function of chronic disease such as occurs in malnutrition. Furthermore, in advanced HIV infection the testes can be invaded by opportunistic infection, e.g. CMV, atypical mycobacteria, Toxoplasma gondii. However, whatever the aetiology, for patients in whom loss of libido is a problem, the administration of testosterone may provide a clinical improvement.

Hypotestosteronism may also result from side-effects of drugs used in the treatment of HIV infection, e.g. protease inhibitors or megestrol. The latter is frequently used for the treatment of wasting and can cause hypotestosteronism.

Indinivar stones

Kidney stones due to crystallization of indinavir in the kidneys is a serious side-effect of indinavir treatment. Kidney stones caused by indinavir deposition are radiolucent (Fig. 135). All patients taking indinavir treatment are advised to increase their daily fluid intake by a minimum of 1–2 l/day in an effort to avoid this, but despite these measures stones can still occur in up to 5% of patients. Patients present with the classical symptoms of renal colic, that is flank pain with or without haematuria. The drug must be stopped, the patient rehydrated and the kidney stones will then normally resolve.

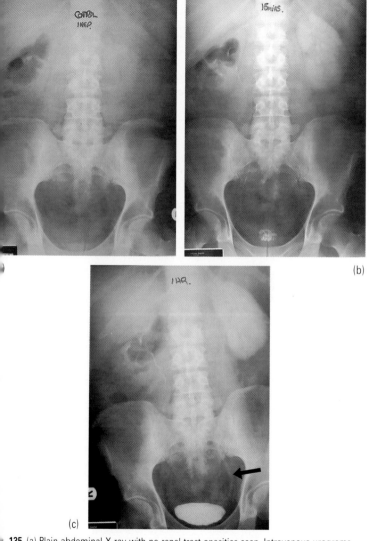

(b)

(c)

135 (a) Plain abdominal X-ray with no renal tract opacities seen. Intravenous urograms after injection of contrast; (b) after 15 minutes—no obstruction on the right side and contrast drains normally; (c) after 1 hour—outline of the entire length of the left ureter consistent with a radiolucent obstructing stone at the left vesico-ureteric junction.

Aetiology

Children are mainly infected with HIV by the vertical route of transmission (see Ch. 19) at or close to the time of birth. Breastfeeding can also transmit HIV. This can be largely prevented with anti-retrovirals in pregnancy, Caesarean section in some cases and the avoidance of breastfeeding. There are a large number of HIV-infected children in eastern Europe, who received contaminated blood or blood products.

Incidence

The worldwide incidence of HIV-infected children may be 10 million or more with an estimated 2.7 million HIV-related deaths by the end of 1997. It was estimated that AIDS in adults had created 8 million orphans by December 1997.

Early signs

Clinical features

Failure to thrive and weight loss (Fig. 136), recurrent diarrhoea, recurrent bacterial infections, protein-losing enteropathy (Fig. 137), poor hair growth, dermatitis and PGL are all common presenting features.

Diagnosis

The appearance of the above features in an at-risk child merits careful investigation. Other causes of failure to thrive and immunosuppression should be specifically excluded. Maternal antibodies may persist for up to 18 months in these children, making HIV antibody testing unreliable before this age. However, a positive test for the virus (PCR for HIV-DNA or HIV culture) after 6 months of age suggests that the child is infected. Persistent hypergammaglobulinaemia may be found.

Prognosis

48% of infected children show clinical signs by 6 months; 26% have AIDS and 17% die of HIV-related disease by 12 months. The median time to AIDS in developed countries is 6 years, and 2 years in Africa. Co-trimoxazole as PCP prophylaxis and the appropriate introduction of anti-retroviral therapy will slow the progression of HIV in children.

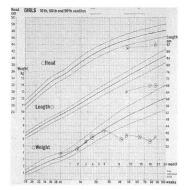

Fig. 136 Progress chart showing decline from 50th centile at 6 months.

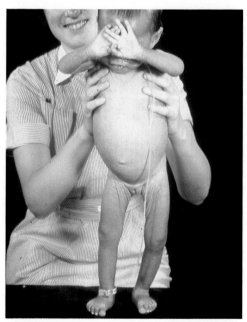

Fig. 137 A child of 2 years with failure-to-thrive. Note tube-feeding due to oral thrush.

Opportunistic infections

Bacteria. Unlike adults, children with HIV infection may have had no opportunity to form antibodies to common bacteria, and so suffer from increased bacterial and mycobacterial infections, such as otitis media, pneumonia and meningitis.

Viruses. Similarly, these children are particularly vulnerable to the common viral infections of childhood, such as varicella–zoster. Viral infections prevalent in adults with AIDS are also seen, particularly herpes simplex (Fig. 138) and cytomegalovirus.

Fungi. Candidal infection is common, and may present as a severe form of nappy-rash (Fig. 139), oral thrush or oesophageal disease (Fig. 140).

Pneumocystis carinii pneumonia (PCP)
As with adult disease, this is a major complication in paediatric AIDS, often contributing to death.

Clinical features

Children may present with unproductive cough and malaise. CXR (Fig. 141, p. 140) is very variable and diagnosis may require lung biopsy or broncho-alveolar lavage (BAL) (p. 111).

Prevention

Prophylactic co-trimoxazole should be instituted in most children and anti-retroviral therapy given when appropriate, according to the viral load and CD4+ cell count. Some US authorities suggest giving anti-retroviral therapy to all infected children.

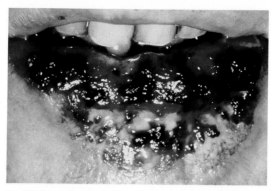

Fig. 138 Severe herpes simplex of lower lip in paediatric AIDS.

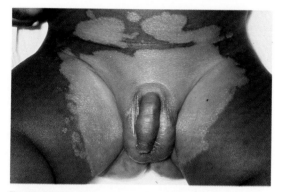

Fig. 139 Scarring following severe candidal nappy rash.

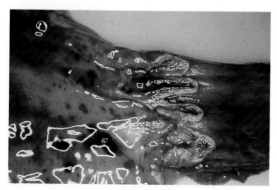

Fig. 140 Postmortem specimen of oesophagus following fatal candida-related perforation.

Lymphoid interstitial pneumonitis (LIP)

Many HIV-infected children develop this condition in which there is extensive lymphoid infiltration of the lung, leading to a restrictive picture on pulmonary function testing.

Clinical features

Failure-to-thrive is common, with progressive compromise of respiratory function. CXR shows diffuse bilateral reticulonodular infiltrates and sometimes hilar lymphadenopathy (Fig. 143).

Management

Anti-retroviral therapy may reduce the incidence and severity of this condition. There may also be a place for steroid therapy and treatment of intercurrent bacterial chest infections, with physiotherapy and oxygen therapy as required.

Neurological disorders

In addition to developmental delay, acquired microcephaly, seizures and encephalopathy occur if anti-retroviral therapy is not instituted early enough.

Other features

Lymphadenopathy and hepatosplenomegaly are often found. Bilateral parotid enlargement (Fig. 142) may be seen. Malignancy is rare in HIV-infected children.

General management of paediatric HIV

Although paediatric experience with anti-retroviral therapy is not as extensive as in adults, there is every reason to believe that the same dramatic improvements will be seen in children. Unfortunately, such therapy is expensive and only widely available in developed countries. Children may now be cared for by local paediatricians with an interest in HIV, with supervision by paediatricians with significant experience of HIV. Careful psychological and social support is necessary. Care may be conveniently provided in family clinics attended by many health professionals.

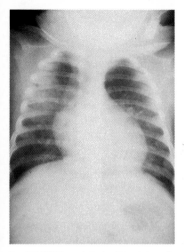

Fig. 141 PCP in an infant, with patches of consolidation in the right upper zone.

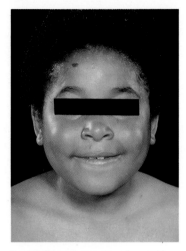

Fig. 142 Bilateral asymptomatic parotid enlargement in a child with LIP.

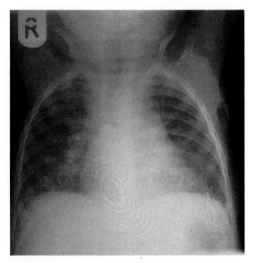

Fig. 143 LIP with diffuse bilateral reticulonodular infiltrate and hilar lymphadenopathy.

The area where perhaps the most exciting advance in the management of HIV infection has been made is that of the reduction of mother-to-child transmission of HIV. In 1999 with optimal medical treatment and the avoidance of breastfeeding, the risk of a baby of an HIV-infected mother acquiring HIV infection is less than 1%. Prior to this, that risk was nearer to 40%. This chapter addresses HIV infection in pregnancy, its effect on the mother and the baby, the role of highly active anti-retroviral therapy (HAART) in the medical management of the mother and baby and in mother-to-child transmission.

Pregnancy itself does not appear to have any deleterious effect on the progression of HIV disease in the mother. HIV-positive mothers do however have a higher incidence of premature delivery and low-birthweight infants.

Mother-to-child transmission of HIV

In the absence of HAART, mother-to-child transmission rates varied from 14–40%. Factors associated with higher transmission rates are listed in Box 5. Breastfeeding can also transmit HIV infection and the risk of HIV being spread by breastfeeding to a previously uninfected baby is about 15%. The time in pregnancy at which mother-to-child HIV transmission is most likely to occur is during labour and delivery. In 1994 following the publication of a study in the USA (ACTG 076), a major breakthrough in the ability to diminish the risk of mother-to-child transmission, by giving zidovudine to the mother (during the pregnancy and labour) (Fig. 144) and the neonate, was clearly demonstrated. By 1998 with the use of triple therapy, by delivering the baby by Caesarean section in certain cases and avoiding breastfeeding, this risk has been further reduced to less than 1%.

Sadly these benefits are less available in the parts of the world where there is the highest prevalence of HIV infection because these treatments are expensive.

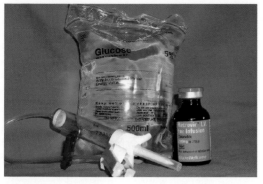

Fig. 144 AZT in dextrose is given by intravenous infusion during labour and delivery until the umbilical cord is clamped.

Treatment of HIV in pregnancy

The decision regarding optimal treatment both for the mother and the unborn child depends on the HIV status of the mother. If the mother is asymptomatic, has a high CD4 count and low viral load (less than 10 000 RNA copies per ml), in the non-pregnant state she would not be prescribed highly active antiviral therapy. However, these mothers will now be recommended daily zidovudine in the third trimester and during labour. As in the non-pregnant woman, if the mother's T-cell count is less than 350/cmm and viral load greater than 10 000 RNA copies per ml, triple therapy will be commenced. In general because of the risk of teratogenic effects, HAART is avoided in the first trimester. The choice of which drugs to use is based on a number of factors listed in Box 6. Those anti-retrovirals about which there is the most data available in pregnancy are: zidovudine, lamivudine, didanosine and nevirapine. Occasional reports of possible teratogenicity with the protease inhibitors have limited their use, and recent reports of mitochondrial encephalopathy possibly associated with the lamivudine/AZT combination have prompted more cautionary use.

Lower segment Caesarean section (LSCS) is recommended if the mother is on AZT monotherapy or the HIV viral load is high. LSCS may not be necessary if the mother is on HAART.

Postnatally, the mother's anti-retroviral therapy is dependent on her stage of the disease. Management of the baby involves continuation of zidovudine for 1 month together with PCP prophylaxis until the HIV status of the baby is known.

Increasingly women who are already on anti-retroviral therapy are becoming pregnant. There are little data available on the long-term effects on the baby or the pregnancy outcome in these mothers.

Antenatal screening for HIV infection

With these advances in the reduction of mother-to-child transmission of HIV, there has been a swing towards universal HIV testing of mothers in pregnancy in the UK. Unless a woman's HIV infection is known about during her pregnancy, she and her baby are denied the opportunity of receiving optimal therapy.

Box 5 Factors associated with high mother-to-child transmission of HIV

Symptomatic HIV disease in the mother
Low maternal T-cell count
High maternal viral load
Breastfeeding
Prolonged rupture of membranes in labour (>4 h)

Box 6 Factors affecting the choice of anti-HIV drug therapy in pregnancy

Mother's prior anti-retroviral history
Mother's partner's anti-retroviral history
Available teratogenicity and effectiveness data on anti-retrovirals
Pill burden and drug tolerability

Highly active anti-retroviral therapy (HAART)

What is HAART?
The use of a combination of three or more anti-retroviral drugs in order to efficiently suppress HIV replication.

Background
Between 1996 and 1999 there was a 75% decrease in new cases of AIDS and AIDS-related deaths in developed countries, largely attributable to HAART. There is now reason to be cautiously optimistic about the future of patients with HIV infection if they can be treated with HAART, an option that is not open to the majority of the world's HIV and AIDS sufferers because of the great expense. At the time of writing, it is felt that a reasonable prospect for HIV-infected patients on HAART is that their infection can be suppressed but not cured. As long as they tolerate medication and are fully compliant, viral replication will be virtually halted, leading to slow recovery of the immune system and a long-term prospect of good health unless treatment fails.

When to start HAART
There is still a debate on this issue which is discussed in detail in various national guidelines such as those for the UK provided by the BHIVA (British HIV Association) on their website at: www.aidsmap.com or the American guidelines can be seen on www.hivatis.org and are summarized in Box 7.

Box 7 Indications for starting HAART in adults from the US and UK guidelines

When the patient is identified during the acute (seroconversion) illness –
  treatment may be continued indefinitely or stopped after 6–12 months
If there are significant HIV-related symptoms
If the CD4+ lymphocyte count is below 350×10^6/l (some use a 500 cut-off)
If the viral load is greater than 30000 copies/ml (some use a 10000 or 15000
  cut-off)
During pregnancy if vaginal delivery is contemplated (see Ch. 19)

Anti-retroviral agents

At the time of writing, there are three main classes of anti-retroviral agent defined by their mode of action, with a likelihood of two more available classes in the near future. The lifecycle of HIV is reasonably well understood and there are many points where anti-HIV agents may act (Fig. 145).

Nucleoside analogue reverse transcriptase inhibitors (NA)

These agents inhibit the RNA-to-DNA reverse transcription step by taking the place of natural nucleosides in the developing DNA chain, thus terminating further elongation of the chain. Zidovudine (AZT) was the first example but other members of this group are didanosine (ddI), zalcitabine (ddC), lamivudine (3TC), stavudine (d4T) and abacavir.

Non-nucleoside reverse transcriptase inhibitors (NNRTI)

These also inhibit reverse transcription, but by a different mechanism to the NAs and therefore there is no cross-resistance between agents in the NA and the NNRTI classes. Examples are nevirapine, delavirdine and efavirenz.

Protease inhibitors (PIs)

Agents in this group inhibit the enzyme that modifies proteins prior to assembly of the virus. Available drugs include saquinavir, ritonavir, indinavir, nelfinavir and amprenavir.

New drugs

These include nucleotide DNA polymerase inhibitors (adefovir and tenofovir) and a blocker of HIV fusin, which is necessary for the virus to attach to cells before entry.

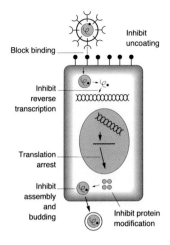

Fig. 145 The lifecycle of HIV showing potential sites for therapeutic modulation.

Anti-retroviral combinations

Apart from the decision as to when to best start therapy, there is still debate about the best combinations to use. Issues to be considered include potency, side-effects, pharmaco-kinetics, ease of compliance ('pill burden') and prevention of anti-viral resistance. There are also certain antagonistic combinations to be avoided, e.g. D4T with AZT. These factors can be complex and require considerable experience on the part of the physician and the patient must be fully committed to therapy. It is wise to counsel the patient about the ramifications of therapy in order to aid compliance in what may be lifelong therapy.

Except in uncommon circumstances (e.g. short-term therapy in pregnancy), current practise is to prescribe three drugs, although four drug combinations or induction (four drugs) followed by maintenance (three drugs) may prove to be the norm in the future. Suitable combinations are listed in Box 8.

Monitoring therapy

The aim of anti-retroviral therapy is to render the patient's HIV levels in the serum to undetectable levels, ideally using an ultrasensitive assay (limit of detection <50 RNA copies/ml). This should lead to a loss or significant reduction of symptoms, prevention of new HIV-related problems and a steady rise in the CD4+ lymphocyte count. This can only be achieved in a fully compliant patient using a potent regimen with a virus that is sensitive to the agents. This may not be achieved in all cases due to poor compliance, poor absorption or other pharmaco-kinetic factors, or if the virus is resistant to one or more agents. Serum virus RNA levels should be monitored at least every 3 months and more frequently if necessary. If treatment fails at least once, samples of the patient's serum should be taken whilst still on therapy for resistance testing (Box 9). It may also be possible to measure serum levels of the anti-retroviral agent.

Box 8 HAART drug combinations

Effective anti-retroviral combinations
2 NAs plus 1 NNRTI
2 NAs plus 1 PI
2 NAs plus 1 synergistic combination of 2 PIs*

Combinations that may prove to be effective
1 NNRTI plus 2 synergistic PIs* plus 1 NA
1 NNRTI plus 1 PI plus 1 or more NA
3 NAs[†]
Any of the above plus adefovir
Addition of hydroxyurea to d4T or ddI regimens

Therapy not recommended
Monotherapy[‡]
Dual therapy
Antagonistic/toxic combinations: d4T + AZT, ddC + ddI, ddC + d4T, ddC + 3TC
Saquinavir hard gel formulation[§]

*Ritonavir plus saquinavir, Ritonavir plus Indinavir, others possible, all at modified doses; [†]Preferably containing abacavir; [‡]Except in pregnancy (see Ch. 19); [§]Except in combination with ritonavir at low synergistic doses.

Box 9 Viral resistance testing

Genotypic testing: RNA sequencing or probing of the main strains of virus in the patient's blood for mutations associated with resistance to certain drugs

Advantages:
Cheaper and quicker than phenotypic testing

Disadvantages:
Presence of mutations does not reliably predict resistance to drugs
Low levels of resistant strains may not be detected

Phenotypic-resistance testing: attempted laboratory growth of the virus in the presence of anti-viral drugs in the culture medium

Advantages
Mimics real life and therefore more likely to be accurate

Disadvantages
Very much more expensive than genotypic-resistance testing
More time consuming – results take longer to obtain
Minor strains with resistance may not be detected

Future therapies

Treatments aimed at boosting anti-HIV immunity, such as with cytokines or therapeutic vaccines, are likely to be introduced in the future.

Additional therapies

Once patients have been established on HAART, prophylactic agents to prevent opportunistic infections (e.g. co-trimoxazole) may not be required once the CD4+ lymphocyte count is above $200 \times 10^6/1$. The patient with an indwelling central line required to administer relatively toxic agents to a near-terminally ill patient (Fig. 146) may become largely a thing of the past.

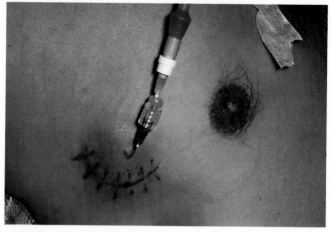

Fig. 146 Central line tunnelled into the subclavian vein for long-term intravenous drug therapy.

Index